What If Medicine Disappeared?

What If Medicine Disappeared?

Gerald E. Markle
Frances B. McCrea

State University of New York Press

Published by
State University of New York Press, Albany

For information, contact State University of New York Press, Albany, NY
www.sunypress.edu

Production by Marilyn Semerad and Eileen Meehan
Marketing by Susan M. Petrie

Library of Congress Cataloging-in-Publication Data

Markle, Gerald E., 1942–
   What if medicine disappeared? / Gerald E. Markle, Frances B. McCrea.
      p. cm.
   Includes bibliographical references and index.
   ISBN 978-0-7914-7305-4 (hardcover : alk. paper)
   ISBN 978-0-7914-7306-1 (pbk. : alk. paper)
   1. Medicine—Miscellanea. 2. Medical care—Miscellanea. 3. Social medicine—
Miscellanea. I. McCrea, Frances B. II. Title.

R708.M34 2008
610—dc22

                                                            2007014885

                        10 9 8 7 6 5 4 3 2 1

For Michael Bruce McCrea
Beloved son and brother

To believe in medicine would be the height of folly,
if not to believe in it were not greater folly still.
—Proust, *The Guermantos Way*, 1920

ACKNOWLEDGMENTS

We thank Allan Mazur, James Petersen and Bob Silverstein for their helpful comments on an earlier draft of this book.

Contents

1

DISAPPEARANCE

in which we pose a sociological thought experiment;
and discuss its intellectual roots, parameters, limitations
and opportunities

"What if medicine disappeared?" I blurted.

"Disappeared?" Fran repeated the question. "What do you mean?"

I was trying to imagine what the world would look like without Western medicine. Gone would be primary care physicians, surgeons, psychiatry—all the various medical specialties. There would be no treatment for trauma, nor fractures. Sufferers from the common cold would need to recover without their physician's help. There would be no blood transfusions or organ transplants, nor would there be emergency or critical care of any sort. Pharmaceutical companies would be gone, as would the drugs they manufacture—as would the placebo effects from those drugs!

Perhaps it was the wine—a favorite bottle from the Rhone Valley—that stimulated my question. Or maybe it was the spring air. Fran and I were just finishing a lovely pasta and homemade pesto dinner on our deck, our table framed by pots of bright red geraniums. As though on cue, a huge heron had flown by moments ago, its wings pumping air in slow motion. In the dusky eve, tree frogs began their noisy chant.

Less poetically, it might have been an editorial in the *New England Journal of Medicine*.

To mark the beginning of the third millennium, the editors of that prestigious, Harvard-based journal, had looked back on medicine's history. We didn't take too seriously their claim that "medicine is one of the few spheres of human activity in which the purposes are unambiguously altruistic." That type of self-serving ideology is pretty typical of any profession—our own included—and easy to dismiss. What got us thinking was the entire point of the editorial—that the history of medicine is a story of progress and great good, that over and above all, the efforts of medicine save lives. "It is hard not to be moved," wrote the editors, "by the astounding course of medical history over the past thousand years."[1]

Who among us, physician or patient, would question medicine's beneficence? Three hundred years ago, Samuel Johnson wrote of medicine that it was the "greatest benefit to mankind," a quotation which is also the title of a recent history of medicine by an eminent historian.[2] Much has changed in the centuries since Johnson. Almost everything about the profession and practice of medicine has changed. But the notion of medicine's beneficence has not.

Earlier that day, we had both read the editorial. We thought about it and expressed some skepticism. But as often happens, we talked around the issue without direction, letting it drift away.

"What if medicine disappeared?" Fran repeated my question. "Probably nothing would happen," she answered with an enigmatic smile.

"Nothing?"

I knew what she did not mean. Were it to vanish, the medical establishment would not go unnoticed. It's a huge part of our economy and our labor force. We spend $1.4 trillion per annum, roughly 15% of the gross domestic product, which comes out to more than $5,000 per capita, double what it was ten years ago. There are 800,000 physicians (up from 300,000 in 1970), 1.5 million registered nurses (double the number from 1970), and about 200,000 pharmacists. In all, our nation has more than four million health professionals.

"What I mean is this, that if medicine disappeared, it wouldn't have much impact on illness and death."

I looked at her.

"Maybe some," she relented, "here and there." She took the last sip of wine. "But overall, I don't think much would happen if medicine disappeared."

The wine was gone. With the darkening, the tree frogs' song turned shrill. Mosquitoes circled, smelling our blood.

After a night of strange dreams, at least for me, we continued talking.

"If medicine disappeared," Fran said, "there are some things we wouldn't miss."

"Such as . . ."

"Such as fatal reactions to prescription drugs."

A trip to the library revealed some amazing stuff.

In 1999, there were in hospitals about two million serious adverse reactions to correctly prescribed drugs, which killed an estimated 106,000 patients, amazingly, the fifth leading cause of death in the United States.[3] By comparison, all accidents in 1999 killed 98,000 people. Lives are undoubtedly saved in hospitals, but they are also needlessly lost there. It seemed that my lifelong fear of hospitals was actually justified.

"What about people who die from infections they get in hospitals," asked Fran.

Back and forth I traveled again to the library, examining 1999 statistics. I learned that so-called nosocomial (hospital acquired) infections afflict about 6% of all hospital admissions, costing an additional $4.5 billion per year in health care expenses, and causing 88,000 deaths—the sixth leading cause of deaths, ahead of diabetes which killed 68,000.[4]

"It many seem a strange principle to enunciate, as the very first requirement in a hospital," Fran was quoting Florence Nightingale, "that it should do the sick no harm."

A day later, Fran handed me a report issued by *The Institute of Medicine*, titled "To Error is Human." The report asserted that medical errors kill between 44,000 and 88,000 people per year (the sixth to the eighth leading cause of death), more than killed by automobiles.[5] Most errors involved the inappropriate administration of medication. Several medical experts challenged the study, claiming that the findings were grossly exaggerated. Yet research in 2002 corroborated the estimate, claiming that "fully 34% of all doctors said that either they or members of their family had experienced serious medical errors . . . with serious health consequences."[6]

Nor is our list complete. To our consternation we learned about surgeries that should never have been performed. In 1974, the U.S. House of Representatives estimated that there were 2.4 million unnecessary operations—a large proportion of them gynecological, resulting in 16,000 deaths and an expenditure of $3.9 billion.[7]

It took us a moment to make the calculation. Taken together, the four medicine-induced problems—adverse reactions to drugs, nosocomial deaths, medical errors, and unnecessary surgery—account conservatively for about a quarter million deaths per year (about one per minute in the United States), about 11% of all deaths. Unbelievably, these medicine-induced problems would be the third leading cause of death, behind cancer but ahead of strokes—though neither alone or together are any of these medicine-induced deaths ever shown in official statistics.

Two nights later we were at our favorite Mexican restaurant, both of us eating entrees that were fried and cheesy.

"So tell me this: How would you evaluate what happened after this supposed disappearance of medicine?" Fran asked me.

"I'm thinking in terms of life or death," I replied, sounding quite dramatic. I took a bite of my chile releno, trying not to imagine my body's response to all the cholesterol that was moving via fork from my plate to my innards. Beginning tomorrow, I pledged to eat more tofu! And to exercise! And to floss! "What I want to know is this: If medicine disappeared, how would it affect mortality?"

"Why just mortality?"

I took a deep breath to compose an answer, but she beat me to it. "Because other ways of thinking about health, such as quality of life, are just too vague, too difficult to assess."

I nodded.

"So you ignore the treatment of pain?"

"Not in real life," I asserted. My wife knew that I had a very low tolerance for pain. "But, for now, yes. Even illness is difficult to assess," I added. "Who knows when someone gets sick or returns to wellness."

"It means, just as one example, that you don't consider the successful treatment of diabetes."

"Sure, I do. But only as it relates to life or death." Sticking to mortality may be a narrow way of looking at things, a laser more than a beam of light. But it had the potential to be revealing.

A day later I showed Fran a quote by Hermann Biggs, founder of New York City's pioneering Bacteriological Diagnostic Laboratory, in 1911, it summarized my argument. "The reduction of the death rate is the principal statistical expression and index of human social progress.[8]

I figured that not much had changed since then. Mortality was and still is the best way to measure the progress of medicine, and yet the physician's task as healer does—and ought to—go far beyond any single way of assessing outcomes.

"What about emergency treatment for accidents?" I asked aloud a few days later. "Without medicine, would a lot of people die?" It occurred to me that our marital conversations had become strange.

"It's hard to know," Fran replied a moment later, "because you can't do any controlled studies."

I nodded. In most spheres of medicine, new practice is certified through carefully designed clinical research. But it's hard to imagine a control group of patients (who get no treatment) in the emergency room, and its even harder to imagine a randomized "double-blind" design (in which neither the patient nor the physician knows who has or has not received treatment).

The next day, we met after work for dinner at our favorite bistro.

"Did you know that the homicide rate declined between 1960 and 2000?" asked Fran.

I looked at her without comprehension. Since I was more interested in addressing my low blood sugar than understanding this turn of conversation, I began to study the menu board.

"But during the same time aggravated assaults with firearms tripled." She paused, waiting for me to say something. "So more people get shot, but fewer die. What's the explanation?"

"Bad aim?" I guessed. I decided to order the whitefish Grenoble. Suddenly it occurred to me. "Shootings increase, but mortality from shootings decreases. It must be the emergency system. There's really no other explanation possible."

Fran smiled. "Mortality from gun assaults has fallen from 16% in 1964 to just 5% at the millennium."[9]

It's like a natural experiment which demonstrates indirectly a substantial improvement in mortality from emergency medicine.

"It's probably the 'chain of survival,'" I proclaimed, "which means that it's not really physicians..."

Here we cannot get one hundred pages ahead of our story. The point had been made. Were emergency medicine to vanish, it appears that more gunshot victims would die—and, we presume, many others with different injuries and traumas would perish as well.

WHY WE DIE

Given our focus on mortality, it is appropriate to begin with an examination of why we die. We all know the litany. The leading cause of death in 2000 was heart disease (30%),[10] followed by cancer (23%) and strokes (7%).[11] The public assumes without question that medical intervention is effective in diagnosing and treating these diseases—and that as a result we live longer. In the chapters that follow, we'll cast considerable doubt on these assumptions and suggest the way that we look at illness and health is wrongheaded. Which leads us to...

A remarkable article that was published in the *Journal of the American Medical Association* (*JAMA*) in 2004. The authors were from the Center for Disease Control and Prevention in Atlanta, a division of the National Institutes of Health (NIH); they were held in the highest regard by the biomedical community. They asked a crucial and generally ignored question: What "actually" causes one to die of heart disease or cancer, or any of the other leading causes of death?[12]

Their answer? The leading "actual cause of death" is tobacco (18%)!

The implications of this finding for personal health and for health care policy are immense. For example, standard medical practice focuses considerable resources on the diagnosis and treatment of lung cancer with very little success. Five year survival rates are about 13%, a figure which unfortunately has not improved in several decades. In an accompanying editorial titled, "The Immediate vs the Important," two physicians, themselves authors of a groundbreaking 1993 article on the same subject, called for a different approach for treating lung cancer. We must begin with the realization, they wrote, that "lung cancer is merely the natural pathologic consequence of exposure to tobacco use." Our ability to eliminate this fearsome disease "will remain constrained until focus and resources are directed to the root causes of these conditions."[13] In other words, lung cancer can be prevented; once contracted, its treatment is most difficult.

According to the *JAMA* article, the second leading "actual cause of death" is obesity (16%).

This is not only a serious problem, but one that is growing rapidly. "Our estimates," the authors explained, "indicate an increase of 76.6% over the 1991 estimate of overweight attributable deaths." In addition to excessive eating, "poor diet and inactivity cause an additional 15,000 deaths per year." By the year 2020, the authors project the leading actual cause of death in the United States will be obesity.

That smoking and obesity account for more than one in three deaths should redirect the teaching of medicine, the considerable efforts of our health care system, and change the very nature of medical practice, for, as we shall see in chapter 8, physicians still give little attention to what are somewhat dismissively called "lifestyle" problems.

THOUGHTS ABOUT THE EXPERIMENT

A few days later conversation about the thought experiment resumed, this time in the car.

"I admit that it's an interesting idea," Fran said, "but there's something suspicious about it." She paused. "It seems like it's just an analytical game."

"A serious game," I replied. The light turned red.

"Because to state the obvious," she continued, ignoring my comment, "medicine is not going to vanish."

As fate would have it, at that very moment we drove by a church, a modest structure with a sign board in front that each week featured a new religious sound bite. *"Imagination Can Be A Dangerous Thing,"* it proclaimed.

We shook our heads. Perhaps that's true, but I prefer the inestimable John Keats, who wrote about the "truth of imagination."

"What I'm hoping is that we can use the 'truth of imagination' to evaluate medicine's role in our health."

"Yeah, sure," she said, a double positive that comes out negative. "Let me ask another question: After this disappearance, what exactly would remain?"

"That's the same as asking me exactly what would disappear."

"Exactly."

It's a difficult question, which, at its heart, involves establishing the boundary—what is inside and what is outside—of Western medicine. The problem is akin to determining, and to maintaining, a political border. There have been frequent wars in medicine's history, and occasional peace treaties, in either case altering a hitherto unquestioned border. What was on one side is now on the other. Maybe the best solution to our problem is to think of what is inside the boundary as the routine practice of medicine, which we would call "MD medicine."[14]

The following afternoon, as Fran was tending to her garden pruning, deadheading, fertilizing, and most of all, admiring her peaceable queendom, we decided that osteopathy, once the bitter enemy of standard medicine, has today become its partner; for our thought experiment, it is part of MD medicine and therefore must be expunged. Chiropractics, on the other hand, is still outside standard practice—even though many insurance companies reimburse its services. We debated acupuncture. It is offered at our local hospital's "Center for Integrative Medicine." Yet it still seemed to us sufficiently outside MD medicine that it would not disappear.

The whole issue of alternative medicine—what its boundaries are and who are its practitioners—is vexing, and problematic for our thought experiment. We talked about an illustrative story.

In 1976, the then Director of the Mayo Clinic Comprehensive Center, Charles Moertel, made a startling disclaimer in *JAMA*. A very dangerous drug, 5-Fluorouracil (5FU), commonly used in chemotherapy for colon cancer, did not—as purported—reduce mortality. "One can only hope," he wrote, "that the good judgment of the American physician will dissuade him from treating thousands of postoperative colon cancer patients with this toxic drug in the misinformed belief that it will provide them with therapeutic benefit."

Two years later, in *The New England Journal of Medicine*, Moertel still maintained that 5FU had no clinical value. Yet he called for continued clinical research on the drug, offering this remarkable conclusion: "Patients and their families have a compelling need for a basis of hope. If such hope is not offered, they will quickly seek it from the hands of quacks or charlatans."

Moertel's assertion was shocking and disturbing.

"We should stop deceiving patients," another physician replied in response: "To do less is to be a charlatan or a quack."[15]

If a quack is one who knowingly gives worthless medicine, then Moertel (along with many other physicians) must be one—a (somewhat facetious) judgment I shared a year later at a symposium I organized at the *American Association for the Advancement of Science*.[16] One panelist, a prominent historian from Emory University, who had written widely on quackery, disagreed. Moertel cannot be a quack, he asserted, because he is using the scientific method in an attempt to advance medicine. In other words, MD medicine cannot by this particular definition be considered illegitimate.

Well, perhaps.

In the years that have passed, we have stopped using the term "quack," except in cases of obvious fraud. Other terms, ones which do not prejudge, better describe those who practice outside the generally approved boundaries of contemporary medicine. But the problem remains: How do we tell who is who and what is what? It's an issue that's still debated.

What ever is meant by alternative medicine, there is no doubt about its widespread use. According to a 1997 survey of the United States, more than four in ten Americans used some form of alternative therapy, an increase from one-third in 1990. Estimated expenditures for alternative medicine professional services increased 45% from 1990 to 1997 and were conservatively estimated at $21 billion in 1997, with at least $12.2 billion paid out-of-pocket. *This exceeds the out-of-pocket expenditures for all U.S. hospitalizations.* Total 1997 out-of-pocket expenditures relating to alternative therapies were conservatively estimated at $27 billion, *comparable to the out-of-pocket expenditures for all U.S. physician services.*[17]

Readers interested in the definition and scope of alternative medicine may consult appendix A. Suffice it to say, for this book, alternative medicine is not seen within the scope of MD medicine.

"What about public health?" asked Fran, changing the subject, just as she crushed a Japanese beetle.

"It has some shared history with medicine," I noted, "and its ultimate goal is similar. But," I listened to myself arguing both sides, "public health professional training is quite different from what physicians get."

A Baltimore Oriole sang to us from a nearby treetop. We craned our necks, but could not find it.

"Its focus," said Fran, "on the whole population, rather than the individual, is fundamentally different." After a moment she added: "In public health, an effect of five deaths per thousand is, and should be, quite significant. But the practicing physician sees one patient at a time. So it's yes or no, rather than a probability equation."

We decided that public health was outside of standard MD medicine and therefore would remain even as medicine disappeared.

The problem of what stays and what disappears is perhaps not as difficult as we first thought. Our criterion of success is mortality. Whether or not the chiropractic or physical therapy or myriad other practices are effective, they have a minimal impact on life or death.

Our previous examples were like foreign wars. But civil wars, that is internal debates within medicine itself, are quite common. The tonsillectomy that I had as a child is no longer done routinely. For two examples since the millennium, hormone replacement is no longer routinely recommended for menopausal women, nor are bone marrow transplants seen as efficacious treatment for breast cancer.

A week later we were still discussing the boundary issue.

I had been wondering how to handle the placebo effect and the whole panoply of mind-body medicine, all of which interested me greatly.

"Most of what we know about placebos comes from clinical trials," Fran pointed out. "If clinical trials disappear, then so does our knowledge, and our understanding, of placebos."

"Sure, that's true. But wait a minute." I found a book, the latest collection of research on placebos, in our study. It took me only a moment to find the quote I was looking for. Most clinicians tolerate placebos "as a necessary nuisance" but otherwise "considered them with contempt,"[18] I read to Fran.

Back and forth we went, often changing sides in the argument. Finally we concluded that the placebo effect, and more generally all of mind-body medicine, has become integrated (if barely) into modern medicine and therefore would disappear.

Extended conversation about boundaries made us realize how, unlike political boundaries, which are lines (or barriers) that one can see and know the instant one has crossed them, the ones that surround medicine are imprecise. This is a problem not unfamiliar to sociologists. Important terms like "middle class" are notoriously difficult to define. Even in medicine, the very fundamental concept of "life" is controversial, that is, to say difficult to define, as witnessed by the fierce debates over abortion and stem cell research, not to mention end-of-life issues.

It's not just doctors and their procedures that would disappear," Fran pointed out. "It's a whole way of thinking about health and illness."

I nodded. Medical practice is more than a set of procedures and techniques. It is directed by a powerful ideology that guides the way physicians think and act. This so-called medical model is based on six assumptions about the body and the nature of disease. I ticked them off in my mind.

First, the concept of health is not defined at all; instead, as in the World Health Organization's definition, it is assumed in the "absence of disease."[19] The physician's task is not to maintain health, but to treat disease, a distinction that has tremendous implications both for clinical medicine and for health care policy.

Second, disease is defined as the presence of certain symptoms and signs. Symptoms, such as aches, pain, or lack of energy, are what bring the patient to the physician's office; signs are objective conditions that can be measured or observed (e.g., vital signs, swelling, fever, cough), through which the physician might discover a disease, perhaps even one unknown to the patient. The objective sign takes precedence over the subjective symptom. Alas, our world is medicalized into an alphabet soup: as we cut into our marbled steak, we worry about its impact on our LDL (low density lipoprotein). At the thirteenth tee, middle-aged men might discuss the advantages of a three-wood as well as their most recent PSA (prostate specific antigen) scores. Thus, does the sign become the focus of attention, the disease, if there is one, being invisible.

Third, there is a clear dichotomy between the mind and the body. Diseases are located in the body and caused by germ or virus or toxin or gene. Treatment involves intervening in or with body functions, or in aiding the body (as with antibiotics) to fend off disease. Even so-called mental illnesses are claimed to have an anatomical, physiological, or genetic basis; this last explanation is in current vogue because of advances in DNA analysis.

Fourth, it follows that disease states are independent from the body and thus cannot really be caused by behavioral aberrations or cultural conditions. The physician treats the malady, not the person. This is called "reductionism," meaning that complex phenomena are ultimately derived from a single principle. For medicine, what this means is that "the language of chemistry and physics will ultimately explain all biological phenomena,"[20] including states of healthfulness and disease.

Fifth, this reductionism leads to thinking of the body as a machine. Each part is evaluated and cared for by a highly trained specialist—blood and skin being parts just like the others. The relationship of one part to another (e.g., kidney to lung), or even one part to the whole, is minimized by the physician's training and the practical organization in the profession. If a part wears out, the physician mechanic repairs or replaces it. If there are problems with the whole, the physician looks for the defective part. We are reminded of a *New Yorker* cartoon, which shows the outside of a suite of physicians offices. A sign lists each doctor with an appropriate specialty, from neurosurgery to hand surgery. The last physician's specialty is shown as "side effects!"

Finally, medicine is a science. The definition, diagnosis and treatment of illness are neutral and objective, unaffected by moral or subjective judgments, or by personal cultural or financial interests. Expertise takes on the highest value, which inevitably means that the physician knows best.

The medical model accounts for, defines, and treats various and sundry human conditions as disease. Over time, more of life's experiences come under medicine's attention. Excessive drinking, treated with powerful pharmaceuticals, is a good example of a behavior that has in recent years been defined as a disease that needs a cure. Various women's issues—birth control, abortion, weight control, breast size, and particularly menstruation and menopause—have come under the "clinical gaze," to borrow Michel Foucault's apt phrase, to be treated with pill or surgery. Birthing is medicalized from conception to delivery.

The medical model individualizes illness, not only minimizing patient input, but also ignoring the importance of the social and physical environment; the food we eat, the water we drink, the air we breathe: these are not taken seriously as causative factors in the patient's illness, or, perhaps more importantly, in the maintenance of the patient's health. The same would be true for the various stressors—unemployment, the loss of a loved one, and so forth—of one's life.

All this flashed through my mind in an instant. There is no doubt that the medical model directs the way we think about—and treat—disease. Without medicine, what would come in its place?

"It's too restrictive," Fran said. "We'd be better off with something else."

"You want to get rid of the medical model?"

She shook her head back and forth. "I want something that includes parts of the current model, but also considers other stuff."

From time to time over the next several months, we would speculate about medicine's disappearance. The snow and cold of a few Michigan winters came and passed. Fran and I, knowing what was best for us, got our vaccinations to protect us from influenza. Then, as we were hard at work on this book, there was a shortage of vaccine. Amidst much public complaint and expressions of fear, many people, we included, were not able to get our vaccinations. Public health officials worried. The winter came and went; we did not get the flu.

Then we got some insight from an article published in the *Archives of Internal Medicine*. Prior to 1980, about 15 to 20% of all elderly persons were vaccinated; by the turn of the millennium, that number had reached about 65%. It was assumed that a health benefit would be conferred on this larger proportion of the elderly. Unfortunately, it turns out that this influenza vaccine bestows no particular advantage against dying from the flu or any related cause. Indeed flu season mortality for older people declined from the late 1960s through the early 1980s. Since then it has remained constant.[21]

Thus, what we expected was not what actually happened. Were a standard medical practice such as influenza vaccines to disappear, the effect on mortality among the elderly would be negligible. The example seemed to illustrate our thesis. Perhaps we actually could assess medicine's performance with a thought experiment.

THREE GIANTS

We are like dwarfs on the shoulders of giants, purportedly said Bernard d'Chartres, the twelfth-century French philosopher. To the extent that he saw further and clearer, he said, it was not because of sharper vision, but rather that he was carried on the shoulders of giants. The phrase has become famous, used by Isaac Newton, and more recently by the eminent sociologist Robert Merton—from whom we learned it—to describe how science advances.

Three groups of giants (for, as sociologists, we always think of groups) have allowed us to imagine this book.

The first group of giants developed the idea of "thought experiments." This is a method of analysis made famous a century ago by physicists like Albert Einstein and Niels Bohr. The idea was to design an elegant experiment, and not be deterred by the fact that it could not possibly happen (trains that travel at almost the speed of light, scales that can weigh one single atom, etc.), perform the experiment entirely in one's head, with as much rigor (and as much pizzazz) as possible, and then imagine the results. In so doing, those physicists revealed some of nature's most incredible secrets.

I wanted to use this same method to get insight about the social world. Readers interested in pursuing this idea—that thought experiments *may be an innovative method* for social scientists— should consult appendix B.

Historical demographers are the second group of giants who have lent their shoulders to us.

Though I'm not old enough to be historical, I like to begin with a memory of my own.

This is what I learned on April 12, 1955: That each summer I would no longer be prevented from swimming in public pools; that innocent children no longer would suffer as did Franklin D. Roosevelt; that the March of Dimes was victorious; that no longer would the first association with the word "Jew" be Julius and Ethyl Rosenberg, who had been executed in 1952; that there was a new hero to worship.

On that day, Jonas Salk announced the successful testing of a vaccine against polio, the last of the dreaded infectious diseases to be controlled. There was a new hero. My family rejoiced. My only problem was that I was supposed to be the one to grow up and cure polio. Now my work was really cut out for me. I'd have to switch my attention and cure cancer.

I did not learn until much later that the celebration over the Salk vaccine was as much myth as science. Yes, the vaccine did work. But what I did not know was that the death rate from polio had already declined precipitously from 1900 to 1955. Surprisingly, the new vaccine accounted for only about 6% of the decline in mortality from polio. Every life saved being the greatest achievement, this is no small feat. Tens of thousands of children would not acquire this dread disease. Yet to focus to closely on the 6% is to ignore the greater lesson from the other 94%.

The polio story was not unusual.

A careful study of historical demography teaches us two things—both quite important for this book—which seem completely counter-intuitive. First, modern medicine has had little to do with the control of deadly infectious diseases, such as typhoid, scarlet fever, and diph-theria.. According to two prominent medical sociologists: "3.5 percent probably represents a reasonable upper limit estimate of the total con-tribution of medical measures to the decline in mortality in the United States since 1900."[22]

Second, modern medicine has had little impact on overall life expectancy. We don't live much longer today than we did at the turn of the twentieth-century. In 1900, a seventy-year-old American, having sur-vived the most dangerous years of youth, could expect to live another 9.3 years. By 1970, a seventy-year-old could expect an additional twelve years, an increased life expectancy of only 2.7 years. This is not an insignificant improvement, but it hardly represents a sea change in mor-tality, especially given the heroic medical efforts often associated with mortality at this age.[23]

Interested readers should consult appendix C for an explication of these unexpected findings.

The third giant was Ivan Illich, a prolific writer, who in 1976 pub-lished the book *Medical Nemesis*.[24] Fran and I had met him years ago when he spoke at our respective universities. He was, to say the least, an impressive character. Illich did not argue that medicine is ineffective. Rather the opposite. Not only that it is quite effective, but also—improbably it would seem at first glance—quite dangerous to society. The first two sentences in his book stated the position clearly: "The medical establishment has become a major threat to health. The dis-abling impact of professional control over medicine has reached the pro-portions of an epidemic."[25] For almost 300 pages, Illich tendered and elaborated these themes. If nothing else, *Medical Nemesis* leaves us with a valuable new word, "iatrogenesis," defined by Illich as "doctor-made ill-ness." For Illich, the medical institution is a great and grave danger to the world, actually causing more illness and death than it prevents.

Medical Nemesis received widespread attention and praise in the popular media. The *New York Times* reviewer noted: "It is obvious that Ivan Illich is on to something here.... Read it and marvel at the light it sheds." Scholarly evaluation was not so positive. The John and Sonia McKinleys dismissed him as a "dilettante." Thomas McKeown wrote that Illich's book has little in common with his own, "except perhaps in the sense that the Bible and the Koran ... are concerned with religious matters."[26] We agree with these critics, for Illich's conclusions shaped his investigation, rather than being formed by them.

Yet Illich, brilliant polemicist that he was, challenged conventional thought and opened the possibilities for critique—and for this book.

TWO SOCIOLOGISTS

Among other things, I study the certification and growth of scientific knowledge; Fran's expertise is in the sociology of medicine. Before reading further, the reader has every right to ask: how objective are the authors? What axes do we have (presumably everyone has some!) to grind? Another wonderful *New Yorker* cartoon comes to mind. "Are you a medical doctor?" asks the skeptical *maitre d'* of the hopeful diner who looks like a professor. "Or are you merely a Ph.D.?" As the latter, are we jealous of "real doctors?"

We are sociologists. By training, we are skeptics of all the professions, our own included, whose members are always (as they should be) influenced by training and vested interests, and whose ideologies are always self-serving. Note that we are not saying that the professions have a negative impact on American life. We don't believe that proposition. Rather, professionals, like everyone else, have certain positions, certain interests, that inevitably affect their behaviors and their views of what they believe to be self evident and good.

Our training leads us to debunk the professions—especially those with high prestige. The very act of writing this book indicates our willingness—our interest—to engage in critique. Yet balanced with that attitude is a real desire to understand the ways of the world for what they are—whatever they are. Our hope is that this book will lead to a better understanding of medicine, and therefore a better idea of how to improve both individual health and the institution of medicine.

Our promise to the reader is this: In an effort to be fair, we will withhold any conclusion until we have evaluated the relevant evidence to the best of our abilities. "The physician," wrote one eminent sociologist, "is not necessarily less objective because he has made a commitment to his patient and against the germ."[27] Yet objectivity, rather than being easy or automatic, "entails some measure of *struggle* in and with the sociologist's self." We hope that this book reflects our struggle.

From both our professional training and personal experience, our attitude toward medicine is deeply ambivalent. Whenever possible, our personal practice is to avoid contact with the medical community. Ignoring expert advice, we rarely give blood or tissue for routine screening. We just don't want to medicalize our lives, at least any more than necessary. Some might call this shortsighted. Perhaps it is, but we try not to dwell on the state of our health. Yet when we do have a health scare, we eschew local service and seek out the very best care available. It is not that our suspicion and mistrust of expert medicine disappears; rather it is that fear of our own mortality asserts itself in the place of intellectual doctrine.

EVALUATION

A few decades ago, authors wrote books about famous doctors. We don't do that. Today, it is common for books about medicine to tell patients' stories, particularly ones with bad endings. We don't do that either. It is also popular these days to write about problems with our health care system, particularly about medicine's high cost, or inequalities in health care delivery—reducing individual physicians "to bits of flotsam on a great economic current," sniffed one editor of a prominent scholarly journal.[28] Our book does not address these issues, though they are of central import to sociologists. Nor do we give much attention to the significant problems of race and gender inequities in health care.

So what do we hope to accomplish?

Almost no one writes about the scientific basis of how medicine is actually practiced. What are the implications of medical practitioners paying too little attention to "W" (e.g., nutrition)? Or of routinely practicing "X" (say, annual physicals)? Or of commonly using "Y" (antibiotics are a good example)? Or of routinely using radically new surgical procedures "Z" (coronary bypass comes to mind). These practices, because they are scientific, are presumed to be off-limits to social scientists.

Yet physicians are not the only ones who can read and interpret scientific literature. Indeed, sociologists—we among them—now study the growth and development of scientific knowledge, from physics and chemistry, as well as biology and medicine.[29] This will be our approach. We plan to examine the very practice of medicine under the microscope. What physicians actually do will therefore be of greater interest than what they think or what others think of them.

Our idea is ironic. For our critique of medicine relies on reports of medical research, written, for the most part, by physicians themselves. Of course, our goal is different from the authors of these articles.

Our method inevitably shapes our book. Our first decision is: which data do we seek, and which do we ignore, in drawing our conclusions? We cannot consider, let alone draw inferences from, stories that begin: "According to my friend..." or "You wouldn't believe what I heard about..." A few moments of watching television, even so-called news programs, demonstrate that anecdotes are commonly used to "prove" just about anything related to illness and health. We ignore all such stories. Even published scientific case studies of one person, or even a few, or even a few score, interesting though they might be, are too limited in scope to help us draw conclusions. Whenever possible, we rely on statistical data. These data give us the best picture of what is happening to most people most of the time.

As much as possible, we avoid coming to any conclusion that is based on a single study—no matter how dramatic its findings. In order for any finding to be seen as conclusive, it must be replicated, preferably more than once. This is the way that good science works. Indeed, according to a 2005 article in *JAMA*, about a third of all "highly cited" papers published in "high impact journals" cannot be replicated. In other words, their findings do not become part of standard knowledge. We should not be too disturbed by this finding, but rather, according to the paper's author, "we all need to start thinking more critically."[30]

In using published research, we understand that not all research reports have an equivalent impact on the profession. Most studies are ignored by the scientific community. A few become quite important. The more prestigious the journal, the greater the likelihood that its contents will become part of generally accepted knowledge—part, in other words, of standard practice. Journals that are official publications of scholarly or professional societies are also influential. Even more important than articles are editorials, which carry the official *imprimatur* of the journal. It is to these editorials that we turn to if and when they are available. One other type of article that deserves our special consideration is called "meta-analysis," or "meta-evaluation," a newly developed statistical technique that attempts to synthesize many different research studies (which often show contradictory or at least varying results) into a single conclusion.

Relying on previously published work creates another problem. According to the U.S. Office of Technology Assessment, only 15 to 20% of medical procedures have ever been evaluated in rigorous scientific trials.[31] The remainder's beneficence is assumed. This is not to say that procedures in this latter category are ineffective. In the wise book, *Lives of a Cell*, Lewis Thomas—dean of medical schools at Yale and New York University and, at the time of his death, CEO of the Sloan-Kettering Institute—claimed that most medical technology is "so effective that it seems to attract the least public notice; it has come to be taken for granted."[32]

Though in this book we argue the opposite, there is surely some truth to Thomas' statement.

For example, approximately 38,000 units of blood are transfused daily. Except for issues of contamination by viruses or toxins, the effectiveness of these 26 million yearly transfusions is not studied. Rather, its goodness is assumed, probably correctly. The efficacy of transfusions is dramatically demonstrated by courts, which on occasion will order the procedure for children even over the objections of parents. A less dramatic example would involve dental care. Almost everyone brushes his or her teeth. Yet we are unaware of any scientific study that establishes the benefit of this common behavior.

There is one more problem with published research. We know that medical researchers, like those of any profession, reflect not only tradition and training, but also vested interests. Therefore most often they will conduct research on problems that they once studied as students. Therefore they are more likely to study problems that will advance their career interests, ones that will allow them to compete for and win large grants—perhaps ones that come from large pharmaceutical companies.[33] As a result, they are more likely to conduct research on chemotherapy rather than on herbal treatments for cancer. It follows inevitably that the body of published research, even with its sample biases, will defend the status quo.

PLAN OF THE BOOK

It goes without saying that medicine and the medical model, at the very heart of American culture, will not disappear. But the very act of so imagining allows us to evaluate its role: for the good—and also for the harm—it does in contemporary society.

Our plan is straightforward. We pursue a difficult—perhaps even subversive—thought: How well does contemporary medicine work? More specifically, what is medicine's impact on mortality? We will guide the reader through a maze of scientific evidence and conclude that of all the human diseases, illnesses and maladies, rather few are treated effectively by standard medical practice. Yet the remaining problems are also treated, mostly without effect, sometimes with great danger to the patient. Thus, it turns out, counterintuitively, that clinical practice and treatment have a minimal impact on our chances of getting sick and our chances of living a long life.

If this conclusion is difficult to believe, we beg the reader's patience. Permit us to make our case.

2

PRIMARY CARE

in which we assess the impact of primary medicine on
mortality, and imagine a world without routine medical
care

We begin with two unremarkable and unheroic, but nonetheless
cautionary tales.

"You have one test result that we need to follow up," said my
internist's soothing voice over the phone.

"What's that?" I spat out after two or three beats of my heart.

"Your PSA, that's 'prostate specific antigen,'" she said didactically, "is
a little high."

I knew something about the test's unreliability, but that was intellectual stuff.

" It's a test we use to detect prostate cancer," she continued, "but it's
probably nothing to worry about."

It all began innocently enough. I had gone to my internist with a
minor complaint, a cough or something like that, probably treated with
some antibiotic, though I don't remember. "When was your last physical?"
she asked. Not receiving the correct answer, she continued: "you really
should have one, if for no other reason than to establish a baseline." When
I demurred, she followed with the punch line: "especially at your age."

A week earlier, I had completed the exam and given my blood. A
week later I repeated the PSA, which once again was high, followed a few

weeks later by several tense days at the Mayo Clinic. The biopsy was negative. Finally I exhaled. God only knows the damage to my health from all the stress brought on by this series of tests.

"See, I told you there was nothing to worry about," said my internist. "I'd strongly urge you to have a PSA test every six months," she concluded.

Which I've done. My PSA is still high.

"I strongly recommend another biopsy," intones my urologist at each appointment. Which I've not done.

Fran's story is similar.

"'Doctor' wants you to take another mammogram, Frances" said the receptionist.

"Why?" She had just taken one.

Fran was irrationally annoyed that the title, 'doctor,' is not preceded by an article. She also understood that as a patient, she had lost her own 'doctor' title and was to be called by her given name.

It had been several years since her last mammogram. At her last Pap test, her (former) gynecologist intoned: "Cervical cancer would be God's punishment for not having had a Pap Smear in such a long time."

As it happened, the routine scheduling took two weeks to the day, followed by four days of waiting for reports to be mailed and then for the phone to ring, during which time Fran worked hard, carefully cared for her flowers, played with her kittens, and worried about dying of breast cancer.

Alas, the repeat test was normal, it being necessitated by a routine blurring—some unexplained technical problem—on the first test. Now, like every other woman, she still worries about breast cancer, but at least not every hour of every day.

The moral to these stories is that we were lucky. Not everyone is.

There is another moral, but to understand that one we need to backtrack and work our way through the system of primary care medicine.

WHO ARE THEY? WHAT DO THEY DO?

If you are sick, or think you need some routine checkup, or a referral to some specialist, you are likely to see your regular physician.

Who are these so-called primary care physicians? They are general practitioners, and a newer specialty called family practitioners, but also included are specialists in general internal medicine. The American

Medical Association (AMA) also counts pediatricians and obstetrician-gynecologists as primary care physicians.

It is a growing—and evolving—profession. In the United States, in 1998, there were 264,000 primary care physicians, almost double the number from 1970. Of these, the most common specialty was internal medicine, 100,000 (41% of the total), followed by 66,000 (21%) in family practice—a specialty that did not exist in 1970. Only 6% listed their specialty as "general practice," a decline of 71% from 1970. Almost half of all primary care physicians were women, compared with 30% women among physicians of all specialties. Among primary care physicians under age 35, more than half were women. Fourteen percent of all primary care physicians practice in rural areas, compared with 9% of all other physicians.[1]

Primary care physicians are well-compensated, but earn less than other physicians. In 1998, the median income for physicians specializing in family practice and general internal medicine was, respectively, $130,000 and $140,000, compared to an average of $160,000 for all physicians—and a high of $240,000 for surgeons (see chapter 3).[2] The income gap between primary care physicians and all other physicians is widening. In 2004, specialists earned almost twice the income as did primary care physicians.[3]

"It's obvious," commented Fran, "that when it comes to money, your family is right! *We are not real doctors!*"

At the turn of the millennium in the United States, there were approximately 824 million visits to all physician offices, which is about three visits per person. About half were for primary care. One quarter of all visits were to general and family practice physicians, which, by definition, would involve primary care. Another 18% were to specialists in internal medicine, 10% to pediatricians, 8% to obstetrician-gynecologists, and 7% to ophthalmologists. Many of these visits were for primary care.[4]

That's a lot of office visits. What happens when you get to your physician's office? We would hope that your interaction with the doctor is thorough and nuanced.

It isn't.

The average office visit lasts only 19 minutes.[5] During the physician's exam, the patient does little talking. A Swedish study found that physicians interrupt their patients' presentations after an average of only 22 seconds. When patients were not interrupted, they spoke for an average of only 92 seconds.[6]

The office visit is not without consequences. Typically it results in an action that continues the patient's involvement in the medical institution. In the United States, the physician orders at least one diagnostic or screening test in three-quarters of all visits, a therapeutic service one-third of the time, and a prescription drug two-thirds of the time. We'll assess the worth of diagnostic and screening tests in a few pages; in chapter 5, we'll assess the efficacy of common prescription drugs

Of all maladies that bring patients to the office, the most common one is the common cold. Its treatment is where we begin.

THE COMMON COLD

In 1994, about one of every ten visits to a primary care physician was for treatment of this malady. In about half of these, the patient's principal symptom was "cough."[7] Other common symptoms were sore throat and chest congestion.

For treatment, primary care physicians prescribed an antibiotic in seven of ten cases in 1994, an increase from six in ten in 1980. For 10 million such visits in 1994, physicians wrote 11 million prescriptions, more than double the number for 1980. In 1999, white, non-Hispanic and younger patients were more likely to receive antibiotic treatment for their cough complaints than were nonwhite and those over age 65. There were no differences between male and female patients.

"All that antibiotic use," Fran mused. "That's a big problem."

She was right. For the most part, antibiotics do not work. The common cold and flu are typically caused by viruses, which cannot be treated with antibiotics. An editorial in the *American Family Physician* recommended "restraint" in prescribing antibiotics for a variety of conditions and began its official guidelines with this explicit admonition: *"Do not prescribe antibiotics for colds."*[8] The guidelines then urged physicians to "develop an awareness of resistance trends in their community."

"That seems clear enough to me," said Fran.

"So why," I asked, "do they continue to prescribe them?"

The editorial supplied the answer. Some physicians continue out of ignorance. Most likely, however, is the notion that few drugs are as "compelling" as antibiotics. "This magic . . . lures patients and physicians alike into the expectation of a quick fix for minor but irritating ailments."

"Magic?" Fran raised her eyebrows. "That's what the *American Family Physician* claims? That's no way to emphasize professional credentials."

Even more. Some doctors blamed the patient for demanding antibiotic treatment, recounting stories of how these customers pressure doctors for prescriptions. What is the doctor to do? "In cases where antibiotics were clearly unnecessary," continued the editorial, "doctors often rationalized their prescribing practices by finding symptoms or assigning diagnoses to justify antibiotic use in order to satisfy the patient."[9]

"So physicians blame the patient for their inappropriate practice," I muttered.

Indeed, both of us agreed that this explanation is disingenuous. It is, after all, the patient who seeks the physicians expertise, and is, a priori, inclined to listen to his or her advice.

Whatever the reason for continued antibiotic use for common colds, Fran and I are distressed. Editorials in professional journals warn against the practice. Physicians, highly trained, must know better.

"It makes me wonder about the role of professional responsibility and ethics in the practice of medicine," concluded Fran. She paused for a moment. "I've had enough of this. My flowers need watering."

Not only are antibiotics ineffective, and indeed in some cases cause severe adverse reactions, but there is also another problem—this one for the public's health. Increased use is responsible for the recent rise in antibiotic resistance among common respiratory pathogens. Current overtreatment, in other words, limits the effectiveness of future treatment not only for common colds, but also for more serious conditions.

The conclusion is clear and twofold: the practice of prescribing antibiotics for common colds and flu is common medical practice, and it is unsatisfactory medical practice, both for the patient and for the public health.

"Maybe Grandpa's cure was not so bad after all," mused Fran.

Seeing my look of incomprehension, she explained.

"As a kid, I didn't know which was worse, getting a chest cold or suffering Grandpa's treatment..."

"Which was..." I prompted.

"A hot poultice of sauteed onions on my chest."

"It probably worked as well as antibiotics," I replied, "and didn't create resistant strains."

"True, but there was one bad side effect," she said, a faraway look in her eyes. "No boys would come near me for several days after treatment."

I smiled, resisting the temptation to respond. Even after all these years I couldn't let my jealousy show.

ANNUAL PHYSICALS

Not all patients who visit their primary care physicians are sick. In fact, most are not. The most common of all reasons to schedule an appointment with one's physician is for a complete physical examination.

This story began in 1922, when, armed with a newly coined medical model, the AMA endorsed annual health examinations. It was based on three premises: that seemingly normal adults can harbor disease; that examination can detect hidden disease at an "early" stage; and, most importantly, that such discovery can lead to arrest, reversal, or cure, and thereby reduce morbidity and mortality.[10] The AMA began a nationwide campaign to promote the practice with the slogan, "Have A Health Examination on Your Birthday." The goal was to achieve 10 million examinations by July 4, 1923.[11]

To promote and standardize the practice, *JAMA* published a manual which detailed a method for these exams. Updated in 1932, 1940, and 1947, it recommended that adults: "Walk at least three miles a day" and "add an orange and cereal to your breakfast." The 1947 Manual advocated the yearly physical as a way of promoting personal vigor and mental fitness. Physicians performing exams were advised not to offer patients promises of good health, but rather to help them modify unhealthful habits.

The life insurance industry, interested in assessing the financial risk posed by applicants, was an early advocate of routine physical examinations. At the turn of the twentieth century, insurance companies began to employ physicians to conduct such examinations. War played a role in the acceptance of this practice. During World Wars I and II, physical exams were used to assess the fitness of military recruits (these exams showed a "disconcertingly high percentage of physical defects among supposedly healthy young men"[12]) and were required annually for all officers of the army and navy.

The practice became common and expedient.[13]

In 2000, complete physical examinations accounted for about 64 million visits out of 823 million visits overall. At a cost of $120 to $150 per visit, and more than $2,000 for the "gold-plated executive physical" that many companies offer to their top executives, that adds up to more than $7 billion per year spent on routine physicals.

What do these exams accomplish?

According to the 1989 *Guide to Clinical Preventive Services*, primary care physicians "have always intuitively understood the value of prevention."[14] Good medicine, in this logic, begins with routine screening of asymptomatic patients, and routine screening begins with a complete physical exam. Indeed, routine screening as part of the general physical examination has been "associated with dramatic reductions in morbidity and mortality." For example, mortality from strokes has decreased by more than 50% since 1972, a trend attributed in part to regular screening for blood pressure, which in turn led to the earlier detection and treatment of hypertension. Mortality from cervical cancer has fallen by three-quarters since 1950, presumably due to widespread Papanicolaou (Pap Smear) screening. Glaucoma, diagnosed in asymptomatic patients, can be arrested with success—though, presumably, this test is done only by specialists (often not medical doctors) of the eye. Children born with metabolic disorders, "who once suffered irreversible mental retardation, now usually retain cognitive function as a result of routine newborn screening and treatment."[15]

These successes are noteworthy. They seem to reveal the value of routine physical examinations of supposedly healthy patients. Yet a few pages after lauding the exam's achievements, the 1989 *Guide* found "inadequate evidence to evaluate effectiveness or to determine the optimal frequency of a preventive service."[16]

Six years prior to the publication of the *Guide*, a different question—with a different agenda— was posed: "How often should a healthy person be examined by a physician, and what procedures should an examination include?" So began a report from the AMA published in 1983.[17]

The very act of raising this question about routine physicals was significant, for it challenged six decades of standard primary care practice. The article was prompted by a groundbreaking report published by the Canadian Task Force on the Periodic Health Examination.[18]

In 1983, the AMA ended a six decade endorsement of a cornerstone of primary care.

In place of annual physicals, it advocated periodic exams, and even then, a minimal reliance on routine testing. The new policy recommended screening not only for blood pressure, weight, and in some cases, breast cancer, but also for conditions that might result from "high risk behaviors."

The routine physical exam is comprised of myriad operations and screening procedures. When these were evaluated one by one, there was little unanimity about either their worth or their cost-effectiveness, and therefore their necessary inclusion in a routine exam. Of course, adverse outcomes are tolerable if the given test has a demonstrable effect on the reduction of mortality or morbidity. The *Guide* urged physicians to be more selective in the use of routine tests.

Perhaps physicians need to adopt a new focus for their practice. The 1989 *Guide* strongly advocated an emphasis on counseling, stating that physicians ought to intervene in the "personal health practices of patients."[19] In the traditional exam, a patient's use of automobile safety belts, for example, would receive less attention than a routine blood screening or chest X-ray. Yet motor vehicle accidents account for 45,000 deaths per year, half of which are preventible by using seat belts. By contrast, "there is little good evidence that performing routine CBCs [complete blood counts] or chest X-rays improves clinical outcomes."

The problem is that physicians are not trained as behavioral scientists. The medical model is, after all, a somatic model. Understandably, physicians are reluctant to trade examination time devoted to soma for behavior modification, which, by necessity would extend the time listening to patients complaints and histories. They are skeptical about the success and cost-effectiveness of counseling; also, according to the 1989 *Guide*, they may not receive reimbursement for preventive services.

In the face of these findings and official recommendations, what is the physician to do? The reduction of death and illness is obviously a criterion in the evaluation of screening. Yet, from the physician's perspective, it would be a mistake to assume it is the only issue. One of the greatest benefits of the patient's periodic visits to the physician is that both have the opportunity "to build the mutual trust and knowledge that will stand them in good stead," not only in times of crisis, but also so that the physician might "foster those behaviors" that contribute to the patient's healthful and productive life. So wrote two physicians in 1980 in the official journal of the American College of Physicians, the *Annals of Internal Medicine*.[20] This is an interesting shift. Not only is the physician urged to counsel, but also work at building a trusting relationship between doctor and patient.

"So let me get this straight," said Fran, crossing her arms around her chest. "I get poked and prodded and humiliated not to prevent some illness or so that I can live longer, but so . . . "

. . . "that you will have greater trust in your physician," I finished her sentence without meeting her eyes.

A 2002 editorial in the *Annals* journal identified trust as a first order goal of the physical exam, important enough in and of itself to justify the maintenance of the entire practice.

> If careful study documents that patients who get annual examinations feel better, behave healthier, undergo more appropriate screening, and *trust their physicians* more than patients who do not have annual physical examinations, skeptics would need to reconsider the value of this yearly ritual.

Direct and intended worth is of course an important issue, but not the only issue. "If low-tech maneuvers, such as listening to patients' chests, engender patients' confidence, we might consider including them in periodic health examinations *despite their lack of proven benefit* on more tangible outcomes." The periodic physical may not only reassure the patient, it might also keep them loyal—prevent them from "falling through the system's cracks"—to the health care system. After this craven promotion of self-interest, the editorial continued: "The regular laying-on of hands and stethoscope (and maybe phlebotomy needle [drawing blood from a vein], too) is not a needless ritual if it fosters trusting clinical relationships."[21]

Thus, we see that the goal of "trust" in and of itself becomes the reason, perhaps the primary reason, for doing—and justifying the routine physical. Other reasons for doing physicals include patient expectation. Consider these two quotes from 2003: "I do physical exams and I do those procedures that lack an evidence base," claimed one physician who is a member of the1996 *Task Force*, "because patients will think they have not gotten their money's worth if there is no laying on of hands." Said another internist: "It's what I was taught and it's what patients have been taught to expect."[22]

"I thought my doctor was a physician, not a faith healer," said Fran.

Her point was well taken. If "laying on of hands" is what patients really need, then faith healing would work just as well—for a fraction of the price. If the practice of medicine purports to be a science—that is, if medical decisions are based on scientific rigor—then this kind of logic cannot stand.

Some doctors still advocate and subject their patients to annual physical examinations. However, as official policy, the practice is dead. But its first cousin, the periodic physical examination, is not—despite a lack of evidence of its utility. In 2003, U.S. Health and Human Services Secretary Tommy Thompson designated September 16 as "Take a Loved One to the Doctor Day." The initiative is part of a program to "close the health gap between communities of color and the general population." With this program, HHS "hopes to generate a greater understanding of the importance of regular health screenings."[23]

A FELINE ASIDE

An odd, but relevant, personal note: a few days ago, we took time out from writing this chapter to take our two kittens, Jekyll and Heidi, to the vet for their routine and "required" shots. A few minutes later we got back into the car, having paid $141, and having declined optional "routine blood tests" to measure myriad baselines, including multiple liver and kidney functions, sugar and hydration, and considered how we might spend the $65 that we thus saved. We carried home, in addition to complaining cats, a printout with our kittens' names, entitled, "*Comprehensive Physical Exam.*"

"Just as annual physical checkups are recommended for people," we read with incredulity, "your pet should be brought in for a comprehensive physical exam each year, even if you aren't noticing any particular problems. Doing so helps us discover potential problems before they become more serious and aids us in keeping your pet healthy." "Please remember," the printout concluded, "an annual physical exam is very important in allowing you to enjoy your pet's company for many years to come."

"Do not do unto others," Fran and I concluded, electing to save Jekyll and Heidi from the benefits of routine pet medicine. Hopefully, our decision was the correct one. At any rate, the cats meowed.

SCREENING

In addition to the "laying on of hands," primary care involves routine screening for a variety of diseases. Following our logic in the previous chapter, we limit our discussion to the two most dangerous diseases: cardiovascular disease, particularly coronary artery disease, and cancer. For each case, we rely on the Report of the U.S. Preventive Services Task Force *Guide to Clinical Preventive Services*, published in 1989 and revised in 1996,[24] and again in 2003.

The 1989 and 1996 *Task Forces* used a grading procedure to evaluate each intervention as follows:

- A=strongly recommends: good evidence, improves health outcomes, benefits substantially outweigh harms

- B=recommends: fair evidence of the same

- C=no recommendation for or against

- D=recommends against: harms outweigh benefits[25]

- I= insufficient evidence to make a recommendation

Interestingly, the meaning of the grade "C" has been redefined in 2003, because of its "location in the hierarchical ranking" which implied that the service is less worthy than ones that receive "A" or "B." The grade "C" now implies that the "net benefits" are smaller than for interventions that merit higher ratings. Such subtle grade inflation results, no doubt, from "controversies sparked by several guidelines," in the words of the *Task Force*. In other words, powerful vested interests cannot be ignored in the preparation of guidelines which have the imprimatur of the government.

That complaint notwithstanding, this chapter could not be written, or not written with as much authority, without these valuable reports. Even if we occasionally differ with the *Task Forces*, we applaud their efforts. We agree with the 2003 *Task Force*, that its efforts are "widely regarded as a premier source of information on the effectiveness of a broad range of clinical preventive services."[26]

Based on our reading of these three works and other scholarly articles, we pose two questions:

1. DOES SCREENING AID DIAGNOSIS?

The simple answer is "yes."

Screening to detect heart disease and cancer do work. *If the goal is to determine the presence of these diseases, then we can say that screening is worthwhile.*

However...

False negatives are a problem. Every medical test, including every screening procedure, has the problem of false negatives—a normal result in a diseased patient.

A good example is the electrocardiogram (ECG). One study showed that three of ten patients with known coronary disease had normal resting ECGs. In many persons, the first sign of the disease may be myocardial infarction or, unfortunately, sudden death. Exercise ECGs (stress tests) are more sensitive, but they are expensive and are also replete with false negatives. Despite these negative findings, the 1996 *The U.S. Preventive Services Task Force* gave a (generous in our estimation) grade of "C" for ECGs (either resting or exercise) for middle-aged adults.

All screening tests for cancer are rife with false negatives. A good example is the PSA test, administered to three-quarters of all men over age fifty in the United States. According to a 2002 study published in the *New England Journal of Medicine*, the much (and, in our view, appropriately) maligned PSA test misses four of five cancers in men under age sixty, and almost two-thirds in men over that age.[27] "Men are now on notice," according to the *New York Times*: "'passing' the prostate screening test is no guarantee that they are cancer free."[28]

False positives are an issue. Every medical test, including those for screening, also has the problem of *false positives*—abnormal result in a normal patient.

Once again, the ECG is a good example. The large majority of persons with abnormal ECGs do not have coronary artery disease and are at low risk of developing the disease in the near future. For these patients, routine screening is expensive and exposes them to risks from more invasive follow-up testing. Office sphygmomanometry (the blood pressure cuff) also produces false positives. One study found that 21% of those diagnosed as mildly hypertensive based on an office test had no evidence of hypertension when twenty-four-hour home recordings were obtained.[29] These false findings are called white coat positives, meaning that the presumed stress of the test itself produces the increased blood pressure.[30]

Cancer screening is also replete with false positives. One in ten mammograms give a false positive result, which leads not only to considerable expense, but also to biopsy and psychological trauma—and even to unnecessary surgery. Fecal blood exam can detect colon cancer, but also produces significant false positives; recommended yearly exams from age 50 to 75 would produce false positives in half of all patients. Various benign conditions of the prostate also produce false PSA positives, leading to considerable anxiety. The best designed studies, which combine digital examination and PSA, show that routine testing leads to needle biopsies on about 18% of the screened population.

False positives are not only a frequent result, but also an expensive one as well. A study of managed care followed routine screenings for prostate, lung, colorectal and ovarian cancer. Of 1087 patients, 43% had at least one false positive. Of those, 83% received follow-up care—which was quite expensive, averaging $1,024 for women, and $1,171 for men. "Along with trials evaluating the health benefits of available cancer screening modalities," the authors conclude, "investigations into potential undesirable consequences of cancer screening are also warranted."[31]

Iatrogenesis is an issue. It is a mistake to assume the safety of a procedure, especially if it is even minimally invasive.[32] Any and all screening that uses radiation increases the patient's risk of cancer.[33] The 1996 *Task Force* admits that radiation probably contributed to "a small number" of new cases of cancer. Such risks may be small for the individual patient, but significant for large populations. Any invasive procedure has the potential for iatrogenesis. Colonoscopy, for example, causes perforation of the bowel—a very serious problem—in one of every 5,000 examinations.

Increased anxiety about breast cancer after false positive mammograms has been observed in both short-term and long-term follow-ups of screened women. Women who underwent a surgical biopsy as the result of a false positive mammogram screening "were more likely to report their work-up as a stressful experience than those who did not have a biopsy." So wrote members of the 1996 *Task Force*, in a statement of the obvious. This anxiety persisted long after the positive test was identified as false.[34]

Stress, we know, is directly linked to the probability of becoming ill and the severity of that illness. While one could argue that a positive test must be followed by appropriate treatment, it is surely the case that a false positive has no preventive value. Rather, in producing stress, the false positive is inevitably harmful in and of itself to the patient. Even worse, a false positive necessitates further tests, which in themselves may be iatrogenic.

Finally, competence is a problem. Would that we could assume competence among physicians. Yet our previous discussion of medical errors—which kill 44,000 to 88,000 people per year—show that we cannot assume any such thing. Like anyone else, professionals included (even professors of Sociology!), physicians make mistakes and have a certain level of ignorance. Unlike other professionals, these mistakes may lead to illness or even death.

Our image of the physician is a person in a white coat, a stethoscope around his (sorry for the sexism) neck. Yet fewer than one-third of all internal medicine programs offer any structured teaching with this instrument. One study of stethoscope use found that internal medicine and family practice residents failed with this instrument to recognize 80% of twelve common cardiac problems, a proportion that was no better than medical students.[35]

Such ignorance is alarming. Surely one would find greater knowledge and competence among specialists. Caveat emptor. According to a study of a medical practice specializing in breast disease, 5% of all women were inappropriately reassured that a malignant lump was benign without biopsy, 3% had a misread mammogram, 1% had a misread pathological finding, and 1% had cancer missed by a poorly performed biopsy. There is a much larger issue here, and one that is rarely assessed. This study, published in the *Archives of Internal Medicine*, a journal published by the AMA, shows considerable incompetence in screening breast cancer.[36] Indeed a 2003 study published in *JAMA* found double the false positives in the United States compared with Great Britain, a finding attributed to inferior mammogram training and fear of malpractice suits. "Very clear and specific standards and targets need to be set for interpretation of mammography," said the study's lead author. "Radiologists who perform outside acceptable ranges need to be told: 'that's not acceptable.'"[37]

We are not saying that a substantial proportion of physicians are incompetent. What we are saying is that the competence of physicians, even specialists, cannot be assumed as a given.

2. DOES SCREENING IMPROVE PROGNOSIS?

The question is fundamental. Diagnosis has value, but not in and of itself. Only when diagnosis leads to decreased mortality or morbidity is it worthwhile. This link cannot be assumed. It must be demonstrated. In the absence of such evidence, diagnosis only leads to increased medical costs, harmful to the economy, to unnecessary and perhaps risky procedures, and to increased stress, which, in itself, is harmful to the patient.

Screening for Cardiovascular Disease

There are two screening procedures that seem to be worthwhile: serum cholesterol and blood pressure. Most medical scientists agree that elevated serum cholesterol (particularly "low density lipoprotein"—LDL) is an important risk factor for coronary disease. During middle age, each 1% increase in serum cholesterol raises the risk of coronary disease by an estimated 3%. Thus, consistent with the medical model discussed in chapter I, we have an important and objective "sign" of health.

Since screening began, there has been a significant decline in heart disease. Yet during the same time, dietary knowledge, especially related to the danger of excessive animal fat, has increased. And smoking has declined significantly. So it is difficult to isolate the direct effect of screening on cardiovascular health, or even on serum cholesterol levels. In one community based study, patients receiving risk factor screening and targeted dietary advice had only 1–3% lower cholesterol than the unscreened controls after a three-year follow-up.[38] The *Task Force* gives a "B" grade for periodic screening of men age 35-65 and women 45-65. There is insufficient evidence (Grade "C") to so recommend for those over age 65 or young adults without a family history of cardiovascular disease.

There is little doubt that lowering blood pressure in hypertensive adults is beneficial, reducing mortality from several common diseases. Small reductions in diastolic pressure (5–6 mm of mercury) could reduce the incidence of coronary disease by 14% and the incidence of strokes by 42%.[39] The *Task Force* recommends with a grade of "A" periodic blood pressure screening for all adults.

There are only two proven ways to reduce cholesterol and hypertension: (1) with powerful drugs (see chapter 5), taken over a period of time, which have significant side effects; and (2) modifications of behavioral risk factors such as smoking, alcohol intake and exercise habits, or dietary changes, particularly decreasing the intake of fatty foods and sodium, or to change life habits with a resulting stress reduction.

The lessons for this book are twofold: (1) drugs treats the sign, not the underlying cause of a problem. Taking drugs may lead to dependency (psychological, if not physical), lessen the motivation for behavioral change, and cause significant iatrogenesis; (2) behavioral interventions are common sense and should be encouraged in all patients, not just those with screening tests suggestive of coronary disease.

Screening for Cancer

The Papanicolaou (Pap) is worthwhile in preventing cervical cancer. A Pap test every third year seems to lower mortality from this invasive cancer by about 91% for sexually active women ages of 20 to 64. The 1996 *Task Force* recommendation for a screening every third year is an "A." There is no evidence that annual screening, a common practice in the United States, improves mortality. Elderly women do not appear to benefit from the test. As we pointed out in chapter I, there is little to say about this important and worthwhile screening precisely because it seems to work and is therefore noncontroversial.

Aside from the Pap Smear test, it is unfortunately difficult to demonstrate the worth of cancer screening.

Lung Cancer. Cancer of the lung leads all other cancers in causing death in the United States. Routine radiography increases early detection, but there is no evidence that screening reduces mortality. The 1996 *Task Force* does not recommend (the lowest grade, "D") screening. They also assign sputum cytology a grade of "D." The entire chapter on lung cancer screening is but three pages in length (about one-quarter the length of other chapters) and offers a grim assessment for lung cancer screening. The implications for our book are clear: *that for this most dangerous of all cancers, medical prophylaxis accomplishes little.*

Colorectal Cancer. For this second most dangerous of all cancers, screening *appears* to improve survival rates. Fecal blood screening could reduce mortality by 15 to 21% over ten years, meaning that annual testing of 500 to 1,000 people for ten years might prevent one death. But at what price? We know that the test is replete with false positives, which cause real stress and suffering, and may lead to further diagnostics with the same result. All this, we should add, comes with significant private and public expense. The American Cancer Society's recommendation— yearly digital exam and fecal blood screening, and signoidoscopy every three years after age fifty—would cost $1 billion annually. The 1996 *Task Force* estimated the cost-effectiveness of screening at about $30,000 per year of life saved.[40] It gave the grade "A" for colorectal screening, concluding that it is "effective in reducing mortality" and is "underused by age-eligible adults."

We are not arguing that lives have prices, but rather that wise health policy must consider, among other factors, cost-effective decisions. Public education about diet or the importance of antioxidants, to cite two examples, might be a wiser investment and accomplish more in mortality reduction than gained by colorectal screening. The implications for this book are not so clear: there is some evidence that screening saves lives. Whether such screening is the most cost-effective approach to saving those lives (as opposed to promoting behavioral changes) is not known.

Prostate Cancer. We pose a story, not so hypothetical. A man has a routine blood test which shows elevated PSA. This finding is followed by a biopsy. Assume almost the worst, that this biopsy is positive. If the tumor appears aggressive, radical treatment is indicated; if not, the question is this: What should be done? Should the patient still be subject to prostatectomy or radiation? The first leads to difficult surgery and recovery; both cause urinary and sexual dysfunction in a substantial proportion of men. These serious side effects notwithstanding, there are other issues. A large proportion of cancers detected by PSA may be so-called indolent tumors, ones that are unlikely to produce clinical symptoms or affect survival. In other words, such tumors may be there, but do nothing that would reduce life expectancy. How does one know if his tumor is indolent or aggressive? How does one make what could be life or death decisions? Perhaps a strategy of so-called watchful waiting is wise, though such (non)action produces considerable and possibly long-term stress with potential negative health consequences.

At stake, in addition to one's life, are the definitions of normal versus pathological. Autopsy studies indicate that most older men, and 30% of younger men (age 30–49) have asymptomatic prostate cancer. One study estimated that 29–44% of cancers detected by PSA were "over-diagnosed" because they would otherwise have been detected only at autopsy.[41] Odd to say, but certain malignancies may be a part of one's ordinary (normal?) life.

A prominent urologist has posed two questions about the dilemmas of screening and treatment: "Is cure possible in those for whom it is necessary, and is cure necessary in those for whom it is possible?"[42] Unfortunately, neither question can be answered at this point in time.

The American Cancer Society and the American Urological Association still recommend an annual digital exam, beginning at age 40. These organizations also recommend an annual PSA for men over 50 (age 40 for African-American men)—at an estimated cost of $12 to $28 billion per year. The 1996 *Task Force* is more cautious, appropriately it seems to us, giving both procedures a grade of "D" for annual screening. "There is no evidence," they conclude, "that screening for prostate cancer results in reduced mortality or morbidity."

There are, it seems to us, two implications for our book: (1) in an unknown proportion of cases, screening for prostate cancer leads, in and of itself, to drastic and debilitating treatment of a condition that may never become life threatening; and (2) there is no evidence that screening for prostate cancer results in any public health advantage.

Breast Cancer. In the city of Shanghai, China, one-quarter million women were divided into two groups. In the first, women were given intensive training on how to conduct breast self-exams, the skill being reinforced one and three years later. The second group received no instruction. Neither group received clinical breast exams or mammograms, which are not widely available in China. A ten-year follow-up on these women published 2002 in the *Journal of the National Cancer Institute* found no difference in death rates between the two groups. These results were consistent with a yet unfinished study in Russia. The authors reached three conclusions:

1. Intensive instruction in self-examination did not reduce mortality from breast cancer.

2. Programs to encourage self-examination in the absence of mammography are unlikely to reduce breast cancer.

3. Women who choose to practice self-examination should be informed that its efficacy is unproven and that it may increase their chances of having a benign breast biopsy.[43]

An accompanying editorial, two University of North Carolina physicians pronounced the self-exam "dead" and urged their colleagues to change their advice to women. Until there is evidence to the contrary, "physicians can stop spending time routinely teaching women's fingers to do breast exams."[44]

The 2003 *Task Force* was not ready to slam the door. "We found no evidence," they concluded, that self-examination "reduces breast cancer mortality." Even so, the *Task Force* gave the grade "I," insufficient evidence, to evaluate the effectiveness of breast self-examination. In light of published evidence, this grade seems generous, to say the least. Such is the reluctance of official bodies to criticize standard medical practices.

We see this same attitude all around us. Last year, Fran attended a defense of a master's thesis. The student, a nurse, had evaluated an educational program to teach women the many purported virtues of breast self-examination. The program worked. Women who participated were more likely to conduct self-exams and, in general, do what their doctors told them to do.

"But does it save lives?" Fran asked.

"What do you mean?" The student's voice was unsteady.

Fran tried to keep her tone nonthreatening. "I know that women can find lumps, but do they live longer?"

"Of course."

"But studies don't show that."

"But those studies are flawed," stammered the student. "Everyone knows that self-examination works," she said, collecting herself. "It's obvious."

It wasn't obvious to Fran. More importantly, it wasn't obvious to the principle investigators of several clinical studies. Indeed, all the evidence was to the contrary.

"Do you agree?" Fran turned to the student's advisor, a Professor of Nursing.

She nodded.

Fran thought about a response. Phrases like "the integrity of evidence-based medicine" came to mind. But what was the point, aside from further alienating her colleagues and leading the student toward a nervous breakdown? Religious beliefs are particularly resistant to proof.

"That's all the questions I have," Fran murmured, studying her notes carefully.

In the student's defense, the American Medical Association, the American Cancer Society, the American College of Obstetrics and Gynecology and the American Academy of Family Physicians still support teaching breast self-examination, and the idea is widely supported by physicians. "The idea that breast self-examination is not worthwhile really defies logic," wrote one gynecologist in 2002. "I've been in practice about twenty-five years, and I have had a number of patients who have found things themselves. In fact, I've had more people find what turns out to be breast cancer on themselves than I or other physicians have found during exams."[45] *Once again we see that the physician's routine practice and local culture are relatively immune to scientific, evidence-based medicine.*

The medical literature on the effectiveness of mammograms is confusing and contradictory. Official recommendations change often. "Is a woman less likely to die of breast cancer if she starts screening while she is in her forties?"[46] This is the question posed by the Canadian National Breast Screening Study. Their answer: Women who received annual mammographies (along with self and clinical breast exams) did not live longer than those who did not.

In the face of this confusion, what should physicians advise women to do? Is routine screening necessary? How often? At what age? The

2003 *Task Force* gave a "B" grade for yearly mammograms for women over forty.

A 2002 editorial in the *Annals of Internal Medicine* maintained that the efficacy of mammograms for younger women is an open question. "The debate is worth following closely," concluded the editor of the journal, "because women are deciding about breast cancer screening, and it's our role to keep them informed as best we can." Yet it is worth remembering that "mammography screening may lead to an overdiagnosis of breast cancer—that is, the detection of a tumor that would not have become clinically detectable in the patient's lifetime." Thus, women must consider the adverse consequences of false-positive mammograms."[47]

Still another editorial (though not by the editor) in the same issue of *Annals* took a harsher view of mammography. "The controversy looks almost Swiftian when we consider that even under the most optimistic assumptions, mammography still cannot prevent the vast majority of breast cancer deaths." This editorial concluded:

> There will come a time when all the study patients have been followed up, all the analyses have been done, all the expert groups have met, and all the editorials have been written, and we still won't be sure how much benefit and how much harm are caused by mammography.[48]

In this book, we are using mortality as an indicator of effectiveness. Thus, the question: What has been the impact of screening—and all treatment—of all breast cancer? The answer: The mortality rate from breast cancer has been stable over the period from 1930 to the present. What this means is that the entire array of *medical intervention*—beginning with *screening,* but also including *surgery* and *chemotherapy*—has not been *effective* in reducing *mortality* from *breast cancer.* This is a very disturbing finding.

Even worse: for reasons not well understood, but at least in part because of earlier and better diagnosis, the annual incidence of breast cancer increased by 55% between 1950 and 1991.[49] Despite our best efforts—huge expenditures which led to early detection and diagnosis, *our efforts to control and hopefully reduce mortality from breast cancer have also failed. This is a significant finding for our book.*[50]

WHAT IF?

What if primary care medicine disappeared?

Ironically, we are not the only ones considering this possibility. In 2006, the American College of Physicians warned that "primary care, the backbone of he nation's health care system, is at grave risk of collapse. The report dwelled on patient dissatisfaction, mostly related to difficulties in timely access, as well as physician dissatisfaction, mostly related to financial issues. Whatever the reason, fewer and fewer medical students are choosing a career in primary care. Between 1997 and 2005, graduates entering family practice residencies dropped by 50%.[51]

What are the implications of this trend for our thought experiment?

When Fran and I first considered this part of the thought experiment, we expected the data would be unambiguous, that losing primary care would lead to disaster, that losing the institutional structure which promoted prevention would have a considerable and adverse effect on our mortality. For if nothing else, we believed in the idea and practice of prevention.

When we actually deconstructed the practice of primary care medicine, the results were disturbing.

There is little evidence that complete physical exams, which are the most common reason for a patient's visit to a primary care physician, have a demonstrable positive effect on health. Few medical authorities would disagree. Some defend the physical exam, claiming that it, or any office visit, creates trust and thus leads to some good. If trust is a means to an end, the argument might hold. As an end to itself, increasing trust is untenable. This argument, which flies in the face of the medical model, is disingenuous.

As Fran said: "It's as if doctors are claiming that their overt treatment does no good, yet interaction with them does, even if they don't really understand how."

Such logic does not bode well for the future of scientific medicine.

What about routine screening? It is not only expensive, but also its results are for the most part not impressive. The 2003 *Task Force* report card is not very good. Many screening procedures are given grades of "C" (e.g., routine electrocardiography for middle-aged adults) and "D" (routine thyroid function tests). For cancer screening, false positives not only cause considerable anxiety, but also generate possible risk from follow-up intervention. Only for cervical cancer is screening effective.

The *Task Force* gives only a few grades of "A" for screening that is routine. In some of those cases, testing often can be and is done in settings other than physician's offices by qualified persons with much less training than medical doctors. Some can be self-administered, such as the blood pressure cuffs at many supermarkets, including one that we frequent (though that particular machine is often busted; when working it often gives results that would make our own mortality imminent).

Screening for all cardiovascular diseases and cancer is usually and appropriately assessed on its effect on mortality and morbidity. Does early diagnosis lead to decreased mortality? According to this criterion, most screening does not do the job.

"Screening also medicalizes our lives," concluded Fran. "We spend too much of our precious time worrying about our blood's level of this or that. We might just be healthier and live longer if we didn't focus on all those signs."

"And false positive from screening cause needless stress. So screening indirectly contributes to ill health," I added.

"And don't forget screening's direct effect on mortality and morbidity from iatrogenesis," she said, having, as usual, the final word.

Thus, the chapter's central question: What if there were no more routine office visits for a variety of maladies, or for complete physical examinations with all its screening procedures?

Such an excision would be significant, for it would deduct some 400 million office visits per year just for the population of the United States, a huge cost savings if nothing else. For persons with conditions that require special treatment, the primary care practitioner acts as a referral agent, passing the patient to an appropriate specialist. For this segment of the patient population, our evaluation awaits analysis in the following chapters. Here we focus exclusively on routine and standard preventive care.

It is not that prevention does not work. Were we to create a world without tobacco (or various environmental pollutants), much disease would be prevented; mortality would be reduced dramatically—not only just to smokers themselves, but also to those around them. As we will show in chapter 8, this is not a hypothetical conclusion. Thus, the issue is not the effectiveness of prevention. Rather the question is: to what degree does routine medical screening contribute to prevention? This chapter has provided some counterintuitive answers.

There is only one possible conclusion to this chapter: Were medicine to disappear, there would not be much of a change in morbidity or mortality.

3

SURGERY

in which we assess the impact of surgery on mortality,
and imagine a world without surgeons

*It is not the fault of our doctors that the medical service
of the community, as at present provided for, is a mur-
derous absurdity. That any sane nation, having observed
that you could provide for the supply of bread by giving
bakers a pecuniary interest in baking for you, should go
on to give a surgeon a pecuniary interest in cutting off
your leg, is enough to make one despair of political
humanity. But that is precisely what we have done. And
the more appalling the mutilation, the more the mutilator
is paid. He who corrects the ingrowing toe-nail receives a
few shillings: he who cuts your inside out receives hundreds of guineas, except when he does it to a poor
person for practice.*

So wrote George Bernard Shaw in 1906 in *The Doctor's Dilemma*.
We had just seen the play at the Shaw Festival in Niagara, Canada. We
laughed, recognizing that like all good humor, the dialogue's fruit had
an ineluctable kernel of truth. At home, we found this gem in the
play's preface.

To offer me a doctor as my judge, and then weight his decision with
a bribe of a large sum of money and a virtual guarantee that if he
makes a mistake it can never be proved against him, is to go wildly

43

beyond the ascertained strain which human nature will bear. It is simply unscientific to allege or believe that doctors do not under existing circumstances perform unnecessary operations and manufacture and prolong lucrative illnesses.

He questioned surgeons' professionalism and their honesty," said Fran. "Which was fair game, and still is."

"But what he did not question was the value of the surgery itself."

Since this chapter's purpose is to consider the disappearance of surgery, this is our very challenge.

WHO ARE THEY? WHAT DO THEY DO?

What is the difference between a surgeon and an internist? asked Richard Selzer, professor of surgery at Yale Medical School until he retired in 1986. "The surgeon, armed to the teeth, seeks to overwhelm and control the body," whereas the internist's approach depends on subtlety. "One is a warrior, the other a statesman."[1]

Like war, surgery has become an important part of our economy. In 1979, there were 85,000 surgeons, a number that increased to 106,000 in 1985 and 153,000 in 1998. Among surgeons, the biggest specialty in 1998 was "general surgery" (40,000), followed by "obstetrics and gynecology" (39,000), which, confusingly, is also counted as a part of primary care.[2]

Surgeons are well compensated, with a median *net (after expenses!)* income of $240,000, the highest of any of the physician specialties. In one online self-report survey in 2002, cardiologists claimed the largest annual income of all surgeons, $475,000 (a nonsurgical specialty, radiology, was next at $415,000).[3]

Once again, Fran and I are reminded of who the *real* doctors are! and are not!

Estimating the numbers and types of surgical procedures is complex. Data for inpatient and outpatient (termed "ambulatory") surgeries are collected separately. The very definition of "surgery" is not always intuitive—especially the newer, less invasive techniques. A spinal tap is not considered a surgical procedure, nor is an endoscopy that does not result in a biopsy—but a catheterization is so counted.

The first estimate of surgery's frequency was not published until 1938 by the Public Health Service and then only for the white population. The most frequently done surgery was *tonsillectomy*, accounting for almost *one-third* of all *procedures* (tonsillectomies are still the second most common surgery on children, and account for one-quarter of all operations performed by otolaryngologists). According to the 1938 data, setting fractured bones was the second most common surgery; appendectomies were third.[4]

In 2000 there were 31.5 million ambulatory surgeries performed, which is 63% of the total operations that year. The most common outpatient surgeries were: 6.9 million for the digestive system, including 1.9 million endoscopies, followed by 5.3 million eye operations, including 2.3 million for cataract removal, then 4.2 million musculo-skeletal procedures, especially in this category 630,000 arthroscopic surgeries.[5]

In 2000 in the United States, there were 23 million inpatient surgical procedures performed, a number which has doubled since 1970. The most common are:

1. Cardiac catheterization—1.22 million

2. Repair of current obstetric laceration—1.13 million

3. Insertion of coronary stent—1.02 million

4. Episiotomy—944 thousand

5. Cesarean section—855 thousand

6. Artificial rupture of amniotic membrane—833 thousand

7. Hysterectomy   633 thousand

8. Surgical repair of fracture—628 thousand

9. Coronary artery bypass graft—519 thousand

10. Endoscopy of large intestine with biopsy—512 thousand

11. Removal of Ovaries and Fallopian Tubes—494 thousand

"What an interesting list," I noted. "With the exception of no. 8 for bones and no. 10 for guts, each of these is either a gynecological or a cardiac procedure."

"*Six of the top eleven surgeries are gynecological*," added Fran, shaking her head.

So it is reasonable to begin our analysis of surgery with those limited to the female population, followed by cardiac surgeries, which comprise all but three of the most common eleven.[6]

GYNECOLOGICAL SURGERIES

Despite all the popular talk about *"natural childbirth," delivering a baby* in the United States is becoming more and more *"unnatural."* In 1980, "artificial rupture of membrane," wherein the obstetrician breaks the amniotic sac to hasten delivery, accounted for only 3% of all deliveries. In 2000, it increased seven times, to 22%. "Medical induction of labor," in which the obstetrician induces labor by injecting a drug, usually Pitocin, increased from 1% in 1980 to 12% in 2000. By the year 2000, these two procedures were used in more than one-third of all deliveries. Add to that the Cesarean section, which accounted for almost one-quarter of all live births in 2000, and we arrive at an amazing conclusion, one that seems to fly in the face of popular ideology: that *six of ten* of all *live births* are induced by some *surgical procedure*—that is, they are *"unnatural."*

Of all major surgical procedures, the two most common in the United States at the turn of the millennium were both gynecological: Cesarean sections and hysterectomies.

Cesarean Section

From 1970 to 1991 the number of Cesarean sections (C-sections) performed in the United States increased 350%. By 1995 they accounted for 21% of all births, increasing slightly to 23% in 2000. This means that almost one of four pregnant women is told either that she is incapable of giving birth vaginally, or that to do so would endanger her child and/or herself. Canada has a similar rate, but in Western Europe C-sections account for only 10 to 14% of all births.

C-sections for severe preeclampsia (pregnancy induced hypertension leading to toxemia), severe diabetes, serious malpresentation, and chord prolapse (premature expulsion of the umbilical chord) may save the life of mother or child. Yet many C-sections are controversial. More than a third are repeat procedures based on the belief that a rupture in the uterine scar may occur if a vaginal birth is attempted, despite evidence that rupture occurs in only 1% of such births. Other conditions where C-sections confer doubtful benefit are dystocia (difficult labor), breech presentation and fetal distress. There are also risks associated with C-sections, most notably for the infant prematurity or respiratory disease and infection. Maternal mortality is two to four times higher compared to vaginal births.[7]

Not all pregnant women have an equal chance of undergoing the procedure. Reminiscent of Shaw's complaint, it turns out that women who are healthier, of higher social class, better insured or cared for in private services are at higher "risk" than their poorer, less-insured counterparts, even though it is lower-class women that have higher risk pregnancies. Hospital stays are considerably longer, and costs considerably higher. Who the physician is also matters. Foreign medical graduates and board certified obstetricians are more likely to deliver by Cesarean; less likely are women physicians and those with professional appointments.[8]

What proportion of all Cesareans are justified? One large U.S. study showed that nearly 40% of all repeat C-sections had no documented abnormalities on the birth certificate to justify the procedure.[9] Most medical scientists estimate that between half and two-thirds of all Cesareans are needless. Two British researchers suggest that a rate of 6 to 8% would be medically indicated, which would save 20,000 surgeries in the United Kingdom and 470,000 in the United States.[10] "It is reasonable to conclude, says health policy analyst Carol Sakala, "that a largely uncontrolled international pandemic of medically unnecessary Cesarean births is occurring."[11] Even eliminating half of all C-sections would bring an estimated savings of $1 billion per annum in the United States—along with, we presume, a significant reduction of trauma and morbidity.

That criticism notwithstanding, the question for this book is: Do Cesarean sections save lives, either the mother's or the child's? In a review of several recent studies published in 2003, the U.S. Agency for Healthcare Research and Quality (AHRQ) found no such evidence. "A higher rate of Cesarean delivery," it concluded, "does not *necessarily* correspond to better outcomes." Pardon our criticism, but the word *necessarily* is not necessary. Delete it and the conclusion is clear: that C-sections do not improve clinical outcomes. "In fact," according to the same article, the rate of C-sections "could be lowered without an increase in infant mortality."[12]

Hysterectomies.

In 2000, some 633,000 hysterectomies were performed in the United States. The rate, which has not changed recently, is double that of most Western European countries. The most common presenting symptom for a hysterectomy is severe menstrual bleeding. Complications from surgery are common: half of all women develop postsurgical kidney or bladder infections, some of which require additional surgery. Radical hysterectomy (including the ovaries) may result in nerve destruction, leading to the inability to control bladder function. In premenopausal women, it also necessitates hormone replacement therapy.

One researcher has shown that a hysterectomy in an otherwise healthy forty-year-old woman increases her life expectancy by some four months, a gain is entirely explained by the 1.3% women who are destined to die of endometrial cancer. For other women, there is no gain in life expectancy; in fact, there may be a decline, given that among women with hysterectomies, there are higher rates of cardiovascular disease.

There are no universally accepted set of criteria regarding appropriate indications for a hysterectomy. Most are done for fibroid tumors that present no immediate problems, inflamation or bleeding, or are associated with abortion or sterilization. One study found that in half of all hysterectomies reviewed, accuracy of the preoperative diagnosis could not be evaluated.[13] Some suggest that a "majority of hysterectomies performed for menorrhagia (excessive bleeding from menstruation) are unnecessary," advocating instead less invasive procedures.[14]

No question: the routine hysterectomy is now under scrutiny.[15] Surgeons are becoming defensive. The title of a 2002 editorial in the *New England Journal of Medicine*—"Hysterectomy—Still a Useful Operation"[16]—says it all.

How many hysterectomies are unwarranted? There is little agreement within the medical community. If we assume 30%, probably a conservative estimate, then 190,000 of these procedures—each involving considerable trauma and expense, as well as some attendant morbidity and mortality—ought not be done.

We should add to this total of unnecessary gynecological surgeries the episiotomy (incision in the birth canal prior to delivery), done more often than either C-sections or hysterectomies. Of these almost one million episiotomies per year:

> There is little scientific support . . . for this procedure. The suggested advantages of episiotomy are challenged easily and the surgery is not without risks. Adverse effects . . . include an increased incidence of severe lacerations, blood loss, pain, delayed healing, dyspareunia [pain during sexual intercourse], psychological trauma and medical cost.[17]

How is all this gynecological surgery to be explained?

"It's not all that complicated," Fran sneered. "It's just a manifestation of sexism. Most gynecologists are males—all of them used to be—and every single patient with a uterus is female."

Fran then told me a story. After telling her pediatrician that she wanted to breast feed her baby, the doctor asked: "for how long?"

"About a year," she replied.

"That's okay if you want to be a cow," he countered.

What she wanted was to be a woman, she thought, but (to her everlasting regret) she did not respond.

That was a long time ago. One would hope that such blatant sexism resides in the past.

But a few hours later, she showed me an newspaper article that she had saved from 1997. It described what was termed a urologist's "prank" in our home state, Michigan. The story is this: a male nurse felt uncomfortable assisting in a Marshall-Marchetti procedure, an operation which requires a nurse to place fingers into the female patient's vagina in order to support the bladder as it is being stitched by the surgeon. This particular urologist dismissed the male nurse for an early lunch and concluded the procedure. When the nurse returned, he was told that the operation was just beginning, requiring him to penetrate the patient's vagina with his finger for ten minutes, after which he was informed about the "joke."

The result: The Michigan State Board of Medicine fined the urologist $1,000 and placed him on probation. A colleague, who was also a member of the Board, abstained from the vote, claiming that "he's a funny guy."

"Not much has changed," muttered Fran, "when criminal sexual assault is dismissed as 'comic relief.'"

In addition to the episiotomy, consider the 494,000 operations to remove a woman's ovaries and Fallopian tubes and the 111,000 mastectomies performed in the year 2000. Most in this latter category are—and have been for at least twenty-five years—controversial. For localized cancers of the breast, it is well-established that removing the lump (lumpectomy) is just as effective and far less traumatic than removal of the entire breast, and perhaps the associated lymph glands (radical mastectomy) as well.

The result of this activity is a huge number of gynecological surgeries of questionable necessity.

CARDIAC SURGERIES

Heart disease is the leading cause of death in the United States Each year, about 1.5 million suffer heart attacks; about a half million do not survive. The cost of medical care and lost economic productivity due to heart disease exceeded $60 billion in 1995. It is obvious that even modest reductions in cardiac morbidity and mortality would have substantial public health benefits.

The underlying cause of most heart problems is coronary artery disease, the most common treatment for which is catheterization or stent. In each case, the surgery involves a small incision in the leg or groin. Catheterization is diagnostic. Its utility cannot be assessed separately from those surgeries which may follow it.

So we begin our consideration of cardiac procedures with the "insertion of stent," a wire mesh tube used to prop open an artery. The stent is collapsed to a small diameter and put over a balloon catheter, which is then moved to the area of blockage. When the balloon is inflated, the stent expands, locks in place and forms a scaffold, which holds the artery open. The stent stays in permanently, holding the artery open.

> *November 22, 2000: Dick Cheney, Vice President Elect, is but one heartbeat away from the presidency. Ironically, it is his own heart that threatens to stop beating, and not for the first time. In 1978 and 1984 he had suffered heart attacks, and he had quadruple bypass surgery in 1984. On this day a few weeks after the election, surgeons install a stent to prop open a narrowed coronary artery. The operation is termed a success.*
>
> *March 5, 2001: The Vice President suffers another small heart attack, this one caused by "restenosis," meaning scar tissue resulting from the original stent—which happens in about half of all cases. The affected vessel is reopened. The procedure is termed a success.*

There is an indirect connection to our hometown, noted by our local newspaper. Dr. Tim Fischell, director of cardiac care at one of our two hospitals, is the inventor of the so-called cypher, a coated stent that releases a drug after its installation. The new stent, implanted in a half million Americans, is intended to prevent restenosis. It was cited as the top advancement in cardiac treatment by the American Heart Association in 2001. The cypher was not the one implanted in the Vice President. Nonetheless the two stories, the Vice President and Dr. Fischell's stent, are covered jointly.

In 2003, the Food and Drug Administration issued two warnings about excessive mortality after cypher implantation. Dr. Fischell denied that the stent posed a health risk. "I don't know what they are doing," he said of the FDA "They must have some other type of agenda." He claimed the investigation was unfair, even bizarre: "The only thing that is strange about this is how amazing this thing is."

Stenting, approved for elective surgery only since 1994, has had an "explosive" growth rate. By the new millennium it was performed more than one million times annually (twice as often on men, compared with women), making it the third most common surgery in the United States today.

Does it work?

Stenting does open blood vessels wider, reducing pain from angina pectoris (literally, "strangling in the chest"). Thus, in the narrow and immediate sense, the operation accomplishes what was intended. But does it save lives? According to a 1999 editorial in the *New England Journal of Medicine*, "it is disappointing that no study has shown that stents favorably influence mortality." In fact, several studies report *higher death rates among those receiving stents*. Remarkably, the editorial concluded that "failure to show a difference in mortality between treatment groups does not necessarily mean that there is no difference."[18]

"That's literally true, but it's bad science," I said aloud. "The burden of proof is on the innovator. One must prove that a technique works."

"Right," Fran replied. "One cannot be required to disprove a negative."

A review of stents in *JAMA*, which sorts benefits into two categories, "proven" and "unproven,"[19] is similarly bad science.

"The logic here is really disappointing," I exclaimed. "There is no such thing as an 'unproven benefit.'"

"Right again," said Fran. "It's more like political spinning than science."

"What's really troubling," I countered, "is that this so-called evidence is being used to justify life or death decisions."

A 1998 editorial in the *New England Journal of Medicine* asked an important question: Why is stenting often performed "without obvious indication?"[20] The editor's answer was fourfold. First, patients and family members insist on "high technology" medical care, eschewing "conservative management" as "obsolescent." In this thinking, the cardiologist has cast aside scientific medicine and medical ethics, and has become an unlikely pawn of the patient. Ultimately, as we have claimed previously, such explanations improperly blame the patient for the doctor's inadequacies. Second, cardiologists simply do not believe the results of statistical studies. What they see from their own patients is what forms their conclusions. Moreover, stenting does relieve symptoms. Ergo, it works. Ergo, we might say, the doctor eschews systematic data for individual and uncontrolled (and perhaps self-serving) observation. Third, "studies that substantiate preconceived notions are likely to be embraced and their recommendations followed, whereas those that do not are often ignored." Once again, the cardiologist eschews evidence-based medicine. Finally, the facilities exist for prompt and aggressive surgery, therefore it can and will happen.

"That last point is like saying: 'If you build it, they will come,'" I concluded.

As an editorial in the prestigious British medical journal, *Lancet*, concludes—with typically English humor: "Stents clearly have a great future—they give excellent predictive results in angiography, are clinically safe, and most of all, *calm the interventional cardiologist*."[21]

"Finally, something I can agree with," proclaimed Fran. "Were I the patient, I would most assuredly want a calm cardiologist!"

Alas, where in these procedures is the fierce warrior? A small incision in the groin is hardly heroic surgery! Our vision of the cardiologist is one who holds the beating heart—and therefore our very life—in his (sorry again for the sexism) hands. This leads us to coronary artery bypass grafts (called "cabbages" because of the CABG abbreviation), more than a half million of these surgeries are performed yearly. In this procedure, the surgeon does indeed stop the heart, and graft a piece of vein (usually the saphenous vein from the thigh) into one or more of the coronary arteries.

Does "cabbage" save lives? The first major clinical trial was in the early 1980s. The Coronary Artery Surgery Study (CASS) consisted of 780 patients who had mild but stable angina. Half were randomly chosen for bypass surgery; the other half received "conservative" treatment. Five years later, 82% from the first group were alive, but 83% from the second. The study concluded: "Coronary bypass surgery appears neither to prolong life nor to prevent myocardial infarction [heart attacks] in patients who have mild angina or who are asymptomatic after infarction."[22] This finding is disturbing, but perhaps we can discount it because of its two-decade age.

In 1987, the National Institutes of Health initiated a study, the so-called Bypass Angioplasty Revascularization Investigation (BARI). In this research, 1,829 patients with multivessel disease were randomly assigned to one of two groups. The first received bypass surgery; the second had balloon angioplasty. The results? For patients suffering heart complications from diabetes, bypass seemed to work better than angioplasty. For all others, bypass conferred no advantage: for patients who received bypass, five year mortality was 4.6%; in the groups that received angioplasty, mortality was 4.2%.[23] According to a 1998 editorial in the *New England Journal of Medicine*: "There were no significant differences for overall mortality regardless of symptoms, left ventricular function, or number of diseased vessels."[24]

Thus, we have two large studies, in which patients were randomly assigned treatment and control categories. Both were unable to demonstrate the effectiveness of bypass surgery. Add to that the increased risk of stroke and the cognitive decline associated with bypass surgery.

"Caveat emptor," said Fran. "Let the buyer beware."

I could only shake my head.

It turns out that stenting and cabbages don't work, but not because of—as previously believed—various technical deficiencies. They don't work because the very model of why a heart attack occurs was incorrect. The old idea was this: "coronary disease is akin to sludge building up in a pipe." Plaque accumulates slowly and irreversibly until one day blood cannot get through a small vessel and the patient has a heart attack. The new idea is that arteries almost never close with sludge, but rather plaque breaks off from any number of places and causes a clot which gets caught downstream, causing a heart attack. Thus, stents and cabbages cannot prevent the formation of these deadly clots.

"I think it is ingrained in the American psyche," said one cardiologist, "that the worth of medical care is directly related to how aggressive it is. Americans want a full-court press," he concluded, blaming the patient for the physician's unscientific judgment. Instead of stenting and cabbages, we would be better off with "boring old advice"; give up smoking, and get blood pressure and cholesterol levels down.[25] Considering these very issues, a *New York Times* editorial concludes: "[we] yearn for the day when there can be much wider testing of one therapy against another to identify those that work best from those that may be oversold."[26]

"Cardiology needs to come out of the closet," concluded Fran.

SHAM SURGERY

From the most heroic to the least: we turn to what is called "sham surgery."

The actual practice of fake surgery is not new. As far back as 1939. a surgeon developed a procedure—ligation (restriction) of the internal mammary artery—to relieve pain from angina pectoris. Three-quarters of all patients reported improvement or elimination of symptoms and the surgery became part of general practice. Twenty years later, researchers found that sham surgery—wherein patients were anesthetized and got chest incisions, but nothing more—worked just as well as those on whom the ligation procedure was actually performed![27]

More recently, a team of physicians discovered that sham arthroscopic surgery (in which the surgeon makes an incision but no instruments enter the knee joint) worked as well as the real surgery for patients suffering from osteoarthritis. Over a two-year period, the group that had the real surgery suffered as much pain and had as much difficulty in walking or bending as did the group that received sham surgery. The *study* calls into question the *necessity* of the 650,000 *arthroscopic procedures* performed in the United States at a cost of $1.5 billion per annum.[28]

How are these findings possible? Sham surgery is nothing more than another (albeit unexpected) manifestation of the so-called placebo effect, which we consider in detail in chapter 6. Yet fake surgery has a very important lesson to teach us.

Concluding this section, we pose two difficult but exceedingly important questions for this chapter: What proportion of real surgeries significantly reduce mortality and morbidity? What proportion of procedures could be replaced by fake surgeries, or by none at all? Whatever that proportion is, tremendous trauma and suffering, let alone huge expenditures, would be avoided.

PREVENTIVE SURGERY

It is the surgeon's task and calling to fix the broken body. The ultimate surgery—both ideologically and financially, for the physician—would anticipate a problem before it manifests itself. Maintenance would replace emergency. This is preventive surgery, surgery on symptom-free patients with the purpose of averting some future harmful condition.

The "quintessential" preventive surgery is carotid endarterectomy. In this procedure, the surgeon removes stenotic or ulcerated lesions at the cervical carotid bifurcation. The intent is to prevent a stroke. In symptomatic patients, the procedure reduces strokes by 5% per year; in asymptomatic patients, the risk reduction is only 1% per year. However, the perioperative mortality is 1.8 percent.[29] In a *JAMA* editorial, two physicians conclude that the procedure "is clearly efficacious in preventing stroke in *selected cohorts* of both symptomatic and asymptomatic patients with carotid stenosis."[30] In emphasizing success in selected cohorts, what is not said is this: that for the great majority of procedures done on asymptomatic patients, the immediate risk is not worth the minimal future benefit.

Next we consider the problem of gallstones, a sometimes painful condition, but one that is not often associated with serious morbidity or mortality. To justify preventive surgery, the benefit must outweigh the risk. Traditional surgery was invasive and associated with hospital stays and long recoveries. In 1989, a far less invasive procedure, called laparoscopic cholecystectomy, was developed. Five years later, it accounted for 90% of all gallstone operations. Case fatality rates declined. There were risks, particularly bile duct injuries, malpractice claims for which increased fivefold.[31]

Enthusiasm for this surgery lowered the threshold for the operation, which resulted in a 22 % increase in the procedure. With more persons now having the surgery, the "total number of gall bladder related deaths in the population either stayed the same or, in some regions, increased by over 10%." A *JAMA* editorial concluded: "It is important that physicians and patients not be tempted into doing surgery just because the surgery now seems easier and because the patient has some symptoms that 'might be related' to gallstones."[32]

Preventive surgery raises serious health policy issues that are significant for our book. The question has been well put: Will "a pound of prevention lead to an ounce of cure?"

> As diagnostic testing improves, more people will be tested. As more people are tested, more will be treated. The spiral of earlier diagnosis and earlier treatment will increase costs but may not lead to an improvement in the health of the population.[33]

Still another example of preventive surgery is quite controversial: surgery to reduce the risk of future malignancy in women with genetic predispositions for cancer. These high-risk women carry one of two mutations, which are carried by 0.1 and 0.2%, respectively, of all U.S. women. Carriers of the former have a 50 to 85% lifetime risk of breast cancer and a 20 to 40% risk of ovarian cancer; for carriers of the latter, the breast cancer risk is similar, while that for ovarian cancer is halved.

Surgery to remove both breasts obviously prevents breast cancer, but it is controversial for three reasons: the trauma of disfiguring surgery, the fact that cancer does not develop in all carriers, and the notion that careful monitoring can lead to effective treatment. In 2002, two articles appeared in the New England Journal of Medicine suggesting the removal of the Fallopian tubes and the ovaries after the childbearing years for such women.[34] Not only would such surgery prevent cancer of the ovaries, which is difficult to detect, it also purportedly reduces the rate of breast cancer.

In an editorial in the *New England Journal of Medicine*, one physician concludes:

> Whether the resulting reduction in the risk of breast cancer, combined with intensive surveillance, is preferable to the more complete protection offered by prophylactic mastectomy is likely to remain a highly personal choice.[35]

Given what is known and what is yet unknown about these mutations, it seems to us that there should be a third choice: to carefully monitor the situation, but to avoid major surgery—which is not risk free—in the absence of symptoms. Note that we are not advocating this third strategy, but rather only its inclusion in the choices available. For reading the history of surgery, we note too many times that procedures are done and later judged to be "unnecessary." Given what we know about doctoring, it is also obvious that "personal choice" is in most cases a sham. What counts most is the preference of the expert physician.

We have another, more general, objection. In those instances where there is considerable family history of breast cancer, genetic screening may be prudent. But we have our doubts about the wisdom of routine screening to detect such mutations. For such procedures serve to further medicalize our lives that are already focused, too much, we think, on the diagnosis and treatment of various maladies. "The more one looks, the more one finds; the more one finds, the more one does." Do we really want our lives, especially as we get older, to revolve around the latest findings from our blood chemistry or biopsy?

Should we not instead seek the *joie de vivre*?

UNNECESSARY OR NECESSARY?

"I've been thinking," said Fran, as she kneaded bread dough. "We've been reading about the term 'unnecessary surgery.'" But what does it really mean? How is it decided what is 'unnecessary'"?

The question is not a new one. At the beginning of the twentieth century, "unnecessary surgery" was defined as criminal behavior.[36] In the 1960s and 1970s, the concept became a product of malpractice case law, with assistance from consumer and women's health care social movements. Litigants were winning lawsuits against physicians for surgical procedures that were deemed by a jury to be needless. In a series of three *JAMA* editorials from 1970 to 1975,[37] the AMA's General Council fretted about capricious juries ("a jury is likely to conclude that the pain and anguish of *any surgery* is worth substantial recompense"), and concluded that unnecessary surgery, "is almost always dealt with as an ordinary case of professional liability based on negligent diagnosis." The offending physician was now characterized (for better or worse) as careless or ignorant, rather than criminal. What is interesting to us is that lawyers, not doctors, came to decide what was meant by "unnecessary surgery."

Some analysts advocate neither the physician, nor the lawyer, but rather that the determination of "unnecessary" be made "by the final arbiter of all surgical procedures, the patient."[38] According to a medical economist, the determination should be made by a "fully informed consumer" who calculates "patient costs and benefits."[39]

For us, the notion of a fully informed patient is sociologically naive. It is the patient who has sought out the surgeon and initiated the interaction, presumably to address some health problem. From the patient's point of view, it is the highly credentialed physician who is the expert. It makes little sense to discard the physician's advice. To do so would fly in the face of the structural power imbalances in the physician-patient dyad. The substitution of "consumer" for "patient" is similarly problematic. Whereas a consumer is free to choose among various retail options, or not choose at all, the patient has initiated contact with the surgeon because, we presume, there is a serious problem. The consumer model (at least theoretically) begins with empowered buyer, whereas the patient's very entre into the system signifies reduced autonomy. This whole line of reasoning comes dangerously to blaming the original problem of unnecessary surgery on the consumer's ignorance, thus, at least in part absolving the physician. In the final analysis, it cannot be the patient who has the major responsibility to prevent unnecessary surgery.

More recently, some have attempted to distinguish "appropriate" from "inappropriate surgery." According to the RAND Corporation, appropriate surgery is

> one in which the expected health benefits of doing a procedure (i.e, increased life expectancy, relief of pain, reduction of anxiety,

improved functional capacity) exceed the expected negative consequences (i.e., mortality, morbidity, time lost from work) by a sufficiently wide margin that the procedure [is] worth doing.[40]

The problem with this definition is that one must begin with a dis-
proof. That is, a given surgical procedure is deemed worthy, or at least not
inappropriate, unless there is proof to the contrary. As we have already
written, this reasoning—disproving, rather than proving—seems back-
ward to us. Even more, benefits and risks are not opposites. In surgery,
the risk is often immediate, the benefit presumably develops over the long
run. The metrics are not comparable. In addition, both risk and benefit
are measured not only by vital outcomes, but also by difficult to concep-
tualize variables, such as those related to quality of life, that are inextrica-
bly cultural. The very term "appropriate" is fundamentally evaluative. "It
implies endorsement of some goal," write two friendly critics.
"Appropriate for what and whom ... to what and whose ends? are questions that must be answered" for the term to be meaningful.[41]

However it might be defined, how much of all surgery is really
"unnecessary?" Consider a technique developed by John Wenneberg,
called "small area analysis." Wenneberg, who holds degrees in both medicine and public health, found that in the 1930s children living in
Oxford, England, were about ten times more likely to have a tonsillectomy than children living in Cambridge. In the 1960s, 60% of children
under age twenty had the operation in Morrison, Vermont, but only
10% from neighboring Middlebury had the same procedure. In the
1970s, the probability of a woman undergoing a hysterectomy in
Middlebury was about one-quarter by age 75, whereas in nearby
Lewistown, seven of ten women had the surgery. In 1982, carotid
endarterectomies were twice as common in Boston than they were in
New Haven, but the rates for coronary bypass were the reverse.
Hysterectomies were more common for New Haven women, but hip
replacements were performed at a higher rate in Boston.

What accounts for these variations in adjacent towns? It is probably
not to be found in the patient population, especially given that Oxford,
Cambridge, Boston, and New Haven are communities characterized by
populations with academic and medical sophistication. It might be
"physician practice style," that relies on the "idiosyncratic clinical decision making."[42] This conclusion seems reasonable as far as it goes. Yet
once again we are suspicious of psychological explanations. We suspect
that something that might be termed "hospital culture"—the local rela-

tions between surgeons and other physicians, the social organization of the hospital, and the policies of the hospital board—is responsible.

What about cities with high rates of surgery? It is possible that its physicians are performing necessary surgeries that save untold lives. In this scenario, the problem is underutilization in cities with low surgical rates. Yet everything we know about the socialization into the surgical profession, the economics of practice, and the sureties of professionaliza- tion leads us to believe that underuse is unlikely. It seems more likely to us—and to Wenneberg—that high rate areas are cities with considerable unnecessary surgeries.

Writing about unnecessary surgery reminds me of my tonsillectomy. Proust was right. When nothing else subsists from the past, the smell and taste of things gain entry "into the immense edifice of memory."

It was a long time ago, but what I remember so vividly about my tonsillectomy is the smell of the ether. "Just take a deep breath," the sur- geon intoned.

It was my first disobedient act against the medical community. I held my breath for all I was worth. But within seconds I understood the terri- ble truth: I had lost. I inhaled the dreadful stuff. Then falling, falling . . .

Then I was awake, puking, too sick to claim my long-promised and long-awaited reward of unlimited ice cream.

Later, in college organic chemistry, the smell of ether always made me ill. That's probably why the class was so difficult for me.

Later still, I learned that my surgery was almost certainly "unneces- sary." Just as every woman with a uterus was seen as a candidate for a hysterectomy, so was every child with a throat a tonsillectomy waiting to happen. Sore throat? Take out the tonsils. No great loss, thought most surgeons. Tonsils don't seem to do anything very important. At the time I lost mine, tonsillectomy was the third most common surgery done in the United States. Today it is understood that these little organs in our throat contribute significantly to the immune response.[43]

The very notion of "unnecessary" often involves cultural as well as medical judgments. For example, about two-thirds of all newborn males are circumcised in the United States. Neither the American Academy of Pediatrics nor the American Medical Association recommend routine circumcision. The procedure does protect against urinary tract infec- tions in the first year of life, and against penile cancer in later life. However, both these conditions are rare. Complications from the surgery itself happen in about one of every two hundred cases, and these are usually minor. Using our criteria of mortality and morbidity, it is difficult to warrant circumcisions. Justifications for the procedure are obviously cultural and religious.[44]

"So 'unnecessary surgery' cannot be defined," said Fran, "without at the same time facing a *subversive idea*."

"Right," I replied, "to define 'unnecessary,' you must first define 'necessary surgery.'"

I watched as she finished kneading. The glistening dough would double in size over the next two hours. I was already getting hungry.

A moment passed. "That's a concept that would make the physician uncomfortable," she said.

"Indeed. Because it raises the efficacy issue *for any* and *every* surgical procedure routine as well as experimental."

"Thinking about those questions calls into question the very mission of surgeons," Fran concluded.

Most practicing physicians define any surgery that is not unnecessary as necessary—two sides of the same coin, a third side not being permitted. Therefore necessary surgery is defined by its negative. Since unnecessary surgery is generally defined by incompetence or malfeasance—the deviant case, as it were—it follows from this logic that the great proportion of surgery is necessary.

There is nothing new about this kind of reasoning. The medical model routinely defines concepts by their absence. Thus, is the concept of disease carefully considered, but perhaps the more important concept of health is not, except by the absence of disease. It follows that health and its maintenance are understudied and poorly understood. This focus on the etiology and treatment of the problematic, rather than the maintenance of the nonproblematic, has a substantial on health care policy. The same would be true for mental health, which is defined by the absence of its supposed opposite, mental illness.

Thus, beginning from a different point, we reach the same destination—that is, the medical model. In a culture such as ours, one that medicalizes the human condition, it will always be difficult to think about, let alone evaluate, the necessity or appropriateness of surgery. Indeed two common surgeries—also cited as the two most "unnecessary" surgeries—are gynecological, no accident given what we know about the medicalization of women's sexuality, particularly related to childbirth. In chapter 6 we will consider a related example, the confusing and unfortunate history of routine postmenopausal hormone replacement.

ORGAN TRANSPLANTS

Some 24,000 major organs are surgically transplanted in the United States per annum, which are about 3% the number of C-sections. Why consider them here? Because organ transplants capture the essence of heroic surgery: highly trained surgical teams, the very latest technology (along with huge costs), and, ultimately, the patient's life or death. Of all major organ transplants, we consider those for heart, perhaps the most dramatic of all, and those for kidney, the most common of all.

The number of heart transplants around the world peaked at four thousand in the mid-1990s and has since declined to just over three thousand per year—two-thirds of them in the United States. Do they work? In the early 1980s, the procedure was new and mortality was high, both from technical surgical and from immune (organ rejection) problems. Progress has been made with both fronts. Do heart transplants work today? There is no easy answer. One cannot conduct clinical trials in which patients are randomly chosen or not for a transplant! Moreover there is a well-recognized problem of selection bias, meaning that relatively healthier patients—ones who would live longer even without surgery—are more likely to be chosen as organ recipients. Yet we know that average survival after surgery is about eight years, which is presumably longer than those who received no transplant.[45]

There were about 14,000 kidney transplants (8,000 from cadavers, 6,000 from living donors) in 2001. Among transplant surgeries, kidneys are the only one for which good alternate therapy exists. Thus, our question is: Do kidney transplants work better than renal dialysis? The answer is an unqualified "yes." For those with transplants there is a 68% reduction in the long-term risk of death compared with those on the waiting list who never receive a transplant. This translates to an increased survival over dialysis of about eight years. Thus, claims an accompanying editorial in the *New England Journal of Medicine*, kidney transplantation should now be viewed as a "lifesaving rather than just a life-enhancing procedure."[46]

In this book, where we have highlighted so much that does not work, treatment for renal failure is worthwhile. Clearly, dialysis works better than no treatment, and surgery works better than dialysis. This is a great accomplishment of scientific medicine.

WHAT IF?

What if surgery disappeared?

The excision would be significant. More than 23 million operations per year would not be done. Surgery's absence would be noted particularly in obstetrics and cardiology. Birthing without obstetric laceration or breaking of the amniotic sac, let alone C-section or episiotomy, would now by necessity happen in a natural way. A variety of gynecological conditions would not be subject to the purported amelioration of major surgery.

Patients with coronary artery disease would not be subject to operations of the heart, from the less invasive insertion of stent to the heroic but oddly termed "cabbage." What would take its place? Perhaps without a purported technical solution, patients—people, that is—would by necessity take more care about maintaining their health through diet and exercise.

Even so...

In a world without surgery, we assume there would be some considerable loss of life, or loss of life extension, or increased morbidity. Most of us know someone whose life was saved by a surgeon, anecdotal evidence to be sure, but data which cannot be ignored. And what of those, perhaps ones dear to us, who have received an organ transplant which improved the quality and quantity of their lives? What about emergency surgery? Were a loved one battered in an automobile wreck, we would not question the need for immediate surgery. Such surgery is the subject of the following chapter.

In this chapter, we have what is probably a sampling problem. Though we have examined the most frequently performed surgeries, we have nonetheless ignored the vast bulk of routine surgery. Are these myriad procedures effective? It is difficult to say. Clinical trials are rare, and with good reason. *The result is that we find it maddeningly difficult to find explicit evidence of surgery's effectiveness.*

Small area analysis and sham surgery raise troublesome issues about the necessity of the bulk of unexamined surgery. The former indicates that a large proportion of operations might be unnecessary. The latter shows that the placebo effect has a hitherto unrealized and major impact where we might least expect it—on surgery, the most somatic of all branches of medicine. Indeed, until we have a greater appreciation of mind-body interactions, we will be unable to evaluate surgery's impact on health. We might go further: from within the logic and practice of the prevailing medical model, it is difficult to evaluate the worthiness of surgery.

Alas, as analysts, we are a part of this world, the one dominated by the medical model. We seek out the physician at the sign or perception of disease. By and large we have surgery when we are told it is needed. Thus, do we enter the institution, signing an inform consent that grants legal permission for the surgeon's cut, exiting only as we are advised, and with the understanding that we will return at the first sign of distress. Our understanding of the institution of surgery is necessarily skewed, not only by available data, but also by experience.

All this being said, and believed, there is nonetheless only one, though tentative, conclusion for this chapter.

Were surgery to disappear, there would be a minimal impact on our mortality.

4

EMERGENCY MEDICINE

in which we assess the impact of emergency medicine on
mortality, and imagine a world without the entire "chain
of survival"

Driving home recently, I had an ordinary experience. I heard the
plaintive wail of a siren. A nightmare—a real one, not a dream—flashed
at the edges of my consciousness. Quickly I realized: Fran was teaching
sixty miles to the north, out of harms way; our children are scattered to
the winds. I exhaled. This was not my problem. On automatic pilot, I
(and every other driver) slowed down, then pulled to the shoulder of the
four lane highway, and stopped. Opposing traffic did the same. The
siren quickened, heightened. A few seconds later, an ambulance hastened
by, its dirge lengthening, lowering, as it sped downtown toward our local
hospital. Normally these incidences have a short life in my short-term
memory. Normally I just keep listening to whatever story is on NPR.
Not that day, probably because I was thinking about this chapter. As I
reentered traffic, and then all day long, I kept wondering: who was in
that ambulance? what happened—life or death? and at some home, perhaps near mine, who might be crying?

This chapter, about emergencies, is different from the proceeding ones.

Our contact with primary care physicians is typically voluntary, or at
least not compelled. We may either have or delay our routine checkup;
many of us postpone our scheduled screenings. We can choose to treat

our colds and other common maladies or wait until they go away—or get worse! Even much of our contact with surgeons is routine, if that word can be used to describe a trip to the cardiologist. A short postponement of an appointment is not likely to matter. Moreover, most surgery is elective; brief delays have little consequence.

None of this is true for emergency medicine. It is completely unpredictable; a moment's inaction may be the difference between life and death.

Our goal in this chapter is to assess the impact of emergency medicine and related specialties on health and well-being. As in previous chapters, our emphasis will be on the impact of this branch of medicine on mortality. *Caveat Emptor*: it is neither possible nor desirable to assess this branch of medicine with controlled, double-blinded[1] studies that we have seen in previous chapters. One can hardly imagine a patient randomly admitted to a real versus a fake emergency room. As a result, there are serious limitations on our ability to carry out our task.

What is meant by the term "emergency medicine?"

At the center of emergency medicine is timelessness and timeliness. The emergency department is open twenty-four hours per day, seven days per week. Definitions of this branch of medicine always include such words as "acute," "urgent," or "episodic." The vital beat must be restored to the stopped or irregular heart; blood spurting from the open wound must be stemmed. Therefore emergency medicine, to a much greater degree than other specialties, is concerned with the moment. And the process: from a "911" telephone call, to the action at the scene of the illness or injury, to the ride in the speeding ambulance—these become crucial life or death precursors to what happens in, and the ultimate success of, the hospital emergency room. By definition, the "emergency" is concluded if and when the patient is stabilized.

In addition to these characteristics, definitions of emergency medicine emphasize the diversity of patient populations, from infant to elderly, from impoverished to wealthy, and the full spectrum of physical (from car wrecks to heart attacks) and behavioral (e.g., attempted suicide) problems. Emergency medicine offers a full range of medical services, regardless of the nature of the presenting complaint, regardless, even, of the method of payment—if there is one.

Whereas there are 264,000 primary care physicians and 153,000 surgeons, there are only 32,000 emergency physicians—only 19,000 of whom were certified by the American Board of Emergency Medicine, and another one thousand certified by the American Osteopathic Board of Emergency Medicine (and 89,000 emergency nurses, 22,000 of whom were board certified).[2]

Why devote an entire chapter to this rather small specialty? The answer to this question rests on the presumption of this book we are concerned about the impact of medicine on morbidity and mortality. Emergency medicine, unlike ordinary day-to-day primary care medicine, is directly related to life or death outcomes.

Or so it would seem.

In 2001, there were 110 million visits to emergency departments (EDs)—a 20% increase from 1992, at the same time that the number of EDs in the United States actually decreased from about 5,000 to less than 4,000. Another way of appreciating this problem: in 1988 the average number of annual visits to a typical ED was about 18,000; by 1998 it was 26,500. In ten years, the ED had 45% increase in patients! One can only imagine the problems this increase created. What ever is going on in EDs, we already know two things: they are more and more frequently utilized, currently accounting for one in ten of all outpatient visits, and they are becoming much more crowded.

How many of these visits were really emergencies?

As it happens, emergency rooms have two separate roles within the health care system. The first is the obvious one, as providers of emergency care. Thus, as in all other chapters, we ask: what actually happens in the ER?[3] and how many lives are saved? The second role of the ER is a safety net provider for vulnerable populations: the uninsured, those on Medicaid, and minorities. The question for this book then becomes: Is this latter function appropriate for the ER? and how does this second role affect the first one?

Let us examine this second set of questions first.

APPROPRIATENESS

The 1986 Emergency Medical Treatment and Labor Act mandates emergency screening, and, if necessary, emergency treatment, at least enough to stabilize the patient for transfer to another facility. The 1997 Balanced Budget Act requires Medicaid and Medicare Programs to reimburse hospitals for what is called "reasonable care." Thus, although it was never planned that way, emergency departments have emerged as "the ultimate safety net for those whom other providers turn away,"[4] as well as "the most important and least recognized federal health care safety net program."[5]

The most frequent visits to emergency departments were from the traditionally disadvantaged population.[6] Those 75 and older, and African Americans, had a use rate about 75% higher than that for whites. About 3% of all ED visits were made by patients residing in a nursing home or other institution. Of these, about three in eight were admitted to the hospital, the same proportion for all persons over age 75.

How many visits are really emergencies?

Of all patients who visit emergency departments, about 12% were direct admissions to intensive care, critical care (see below) or a coronary unit. This does not mean that the other 88% are not emergencies. In 1.5% of all cases, the patient leaves the emergency room without seeing a physician. One of ten see a doctor, but no follow-up is planned; two of five are referred to another doctor or clinic for a follow-up. In itself, this tells us little. Quite possibly, a patient presents himself or herself with an open wound, which might be cleaned and sutured. Such a person, bleeding upon presentation, surely needed immediate care, but did not need extended care via hospitalization.[7]

Still, our question is unanswered.

Triage tells us more. At intake, patients' problems are assigned a level of immediacy. Beginning in 1990, patients who needed immediate care, within 15 minutes, were termed "emergent." Those deemed "urgent" need to be treated within the hour; all others were labeled "nonurgent," defined as "not life or limb threatening." Nonurgent patients "probably could be treated in a doctors office or clinic." According to a 1990 study by the U.S. General Accounting Office (GAO), fully 43% of all emergency visits were nonurgent.[8]

The most recent data, for 2001, was published in 2003, by the National Center for Health Statistics. It shows that 19% of all visits are "emergent" and 32% are "urgent." Next, most interestingly, *a new* category *has been added: 16% are* deemed *"semi-urgent," defined* as *patients who should be seen* within *1–2 hours*! Alas, according to this classification, only 9% of all visits are "non-urgent."[9]

"It appears that medicine and politics are sharing the same hospital bed!" I said, catching my breath. We were raking leaves, and it annoyed me that I tired much more quickly than she did.

"What's new about that," Fran replied, continuing the job at hand.

It would seem that this new category, "semi-urgent," is misleading. Clearly for them there is no danger of life or limb. It would seem prudent (but not politically expedient) to once again combine this group with "nonurgent."

There is yet another issue in the interpretation of the data. In about one-quarter of all cases, triage—for reasons unknown or unspecified—is not performed. It seems commonsensical (and conservative) to apportion without bias this group into the other four categories. Thus 9% of this group can be assumed to be nonurgent and another 16% semi-urgent.

"So according to this recalculation," said Fran, "at least one-third of all emergency visits are nonurgent."

"And I was reading earlier that those classified as nonurgent are disproportionally young adult African Americans." I gathered my jacket around me. There was a chill in the air.

"That's the tip of a yet another problem," she concluded.

Alas, when all is said and done, we do not know the proportion of all visits to emergency rooms that are indeed emergencies. The most recent government statistics would have us believe that only about one in ten are nonurgent. *Our best guess would be somewhere between one-third and one-half.*

So what is the problem? Is "nonurgent" the same as "inappropriate?" Is it wrong to have a medical safety net—a place where medical care is a civil right extended to all?

One problem is cost. In a 1993 speech before a joint session of Congress, President Bill Clinton targeted nonurgent emergency visits for cost reduction. Typically such visits are five times more costly than comparable visits to a clinic or a physician's office. But are they inappropriate? The physician's office or the clinic may be closed, or they may choose not to treat the perspective patient. Indeed, from the prospective of an individual with limited resources, the emergency department may be the only option. A nonurgent visit may be far more appropriate (and prudent) than seeking no care at all.

Moreover, ER cost might be deceptive. In fact, in 1996 emergency department expenditures accounted for only 1.9% of the total national health expenditure.[10] In all, "the potential savings from a diversion of nonurgent visits to private physician's offices may be much less than it is widely believed."[11]

What we are saying is this: it makes little sense for EDs to function as safety nets; surely one could design more rational—convenient and cost-effective—systems. Indeed, many hospitals have closed their emergency rooms; others turn away ambulances or "dump" patients who require critical care and cannot pay—leading to what one critic calls "no room at the inn."[12] Still other hospitals have cut available emergency room services, resulting in long waiting lines.

We have completed our consideration related to the second function of EDs—that is, as a medical safety net. We turn now to an assessment of emergency medicine's efficacy for those who have medical problems, perhaps life-and-death problems.

LIFE OR DEATH?

Of course, not all ER visits are for life or death problems. In 2001, the most common reason for a visit—one of every three—was for poisoning or injury (especially as a result of alcohol use)—the two being categorized together); next, one of eight visits, was for acute upper respiratory infection. Adverse reaction to drugs (alas, no distinction is made between legal, prescription drugs, and illegal ones) accounted for about one in thirteen of all ED admissions.

For these various and sundry problems, about 85% of all patients receive some sort of diagnostic or screening service. The most common tests are blood work, done about half the time, followed by X-rays in two of five admissions. The use of CAT scans and magnetic resonance imaging (MRI) has almost tripled in the past ten years; 6% of all patients now receive one or the other diagnostic—a statistic that will merit attention in our concluding chapter.

Three of four admissions received some sort of medication. The most common medications were for pain relief, the most prescribed being acetaminophen (Tylenol) and ibuprofen (Advil) perhaps an indication of seriousness, or lack thereof. The third most often prescribed drug (8.1 million for emergency visits in 2000) was hydrocodone, mostly under the brand name, Vicodin. This drug is a powerful and addictive semisynthetic narcotic. In the chapter that follows, we will consider its appropriate (and inappropriate) uses. Taken together, pain relievers accounted for one-third of all medications. The next most category of drugs (15%) were antibiotics, the overprescription of which, documented in the preceding chapter, is a significant public health problem.

Only one in twenty patients arrive at the emergency room with that most fearsome symptom—chest pain—as their primary symptom, though heart problems are the most common ED physician diagnosis among those over age 45. Although the number of patients is relatively small, the potential consequences of chest pain are life or death.

Sudden cardiac arrest is the number one killer of adults in the United States. Each year, about one-quarter million die suddenly, often with no symptom onset. If cardiac arrest happens to a patient already in the hospital, the survival rate in the United States is about 15%. A study in Australia showed that an emergency medical team within a hospital could respond to "physiological instabilities" that precede most such attacks, and decrease the actual incidence of cardiac arrest by about two-thirds, and therefore substantially reduce the death rate.[13]

Prior to arrival at the hospital, resuscitation after cardiac arrest is possible, but only with what is termed "the chain of survival": quick access to emergency care, cardiopulmonary resuscitation (CPR), defibrillation, and advanced care. Each of the four is necessary; moreover, it is crucial that the sequencing be rapid. If possible, CPR should be performed by a bystander. Indeed, a meta-analysis of 37 studies found that a 5% increment in bystander CPR is associated with an absolute increase in survival of 0.3% to 1%—a small, but significant decrease in mortality.[14]

One study in 1979 found that when CPR is started within four minutes of collapse, and when advanced care is instituted within eight minutes, the survival to hospital discharge was 43%.[15] Other studies have confirmed the importance of the "chain of survival," though with less dramatic results.

Reading these research reports, we lamented the fact that neither of us knows how to administer CPR.

"It's simple to learn and simple to do," said Fran.

"That's true, but it doesn't work very well," I rationalized.

Our real resistance had a different origin with the realization it would force on us yet another glimpses of our own, and each other's, mortality.

"As soon as we have the time, let's take lessons," said Fran.

"The Red Cross would be a good place."

Fran nodded. "Maybe when this book is completed."

Our hands were over our hearts, but not to pledge allegiance.

A 2003 study of Seattle and its surrounding area found that without emergency service intervention, not one of 2,277 people survived what were termed such "death events." With timely emergency care (e.g., oxygen, aspirin, beta-blockers, nitrates, antiarrhythmic agents, and, of course, quick hospital transport) 128 of 1428—that is, 9%—survived. This improvement in mortality—saving these lives—is surely impressive.[16]

Within the "chain of survival," research shows the particular importance of early defibrillation. A study of 19 urban and suburban communities in

Ontario, Canada, found that firefighters were able to reach 90% of all patients with cardiac arrest in eight minutes. Following the introduction of defibrillators used on several thousand patients, survival increased from 3.9% to 5.2%.[17] Another study showed that with each minute defibrillation is delayed, the chances of successful resuscitation decrease anywhere from 2% to 10%.[18]

While such improvement is laudable—each life saved being precious—it is obvious that most people who suffer cardiac arrest die.

Because defibrillators seem to work (although, again, the effect is not that great), and because they are relatively inexpensive, there have been considerable efforts to make them available in as many public places as possible. In an interesting study of a casino in Windsor, Ontario, there were 23 cases of cardiac arrest in a five-year period, from 1994 to 1999. All were witnessed on videotape. The casino was equipped with defibrillators. Average time to initial defibrillation was 7.7 minutes; average time for EMS to arrive was 13.3 minutes. Fifteen of the twenty-three patients—almost two of three—were discharged alive from the hospital. During the same time period, 668 patients experienced cardiac arrest in the greater Windsor community. Only 37 (5.5%) survived.[19]

Reading this research we may conclude that defibrillators surely are effective. But is the lifesaving effect a little or a lot? We just don't know. Whatever the effect, it would appear wise to equip all public places with defibrillators. One problem: only 16% of all cardiac arrests happen in public places. So even a widespread program to make this equipment available, and train people in their use, would have a minimal effect on survival—especially given this technology's marginal effect on mortality.

Some have proposed that high-risk patients be allowed to purchase portable home defibrillators. Currently this is not permissible under law. Moreover, such equipment would cost several thousand dollars, though most agree that this price could come down with volume sales.

Even if the marginal gains are not huge, why not spend the money?

In reality, the choice is usually not whether to spend, but what to spend it on. Given the choice of spending $1,500 to purchase a home defibrillator, "or spending a comparable amount of money on a bicycle, a smoking cessation program, a health club membership, or treatment of hypertension," writes one skeptic, "most people would be better served by choosing one of the latter for themselves or a loved one."[20]

As profound skeptics of medicalization, we agree. We would add that the cash could be spent, perhaps more wisely—and could perhaps promote better health—for a vacation, mountain or sea, depending upon one's preferences.

In our assessment of emergency medicine, one more issue must be addressed. As we have seen in previous chapters, mistakes in all branches of medicine—as in all branches of life—are made. Some patients are incorrectly diagnosed. According to one study of ten emergency rooms, 2% of patients with acute myocardial infarction (serious heart attacks)—and another 2% with unstable angina (a precursor to serious heart attacks)—were inappropriately discharged.[21] Each one of these mistakes is reprehensible; each must be understood, and in so doing, effort must be made to avoid further errors. Having said that, we do not and cannot live in a society without error. Heart disease may have an array of presenting symptoms, and therefore a success rate of 98% should not be too quickly criticized.

One important cautionary note about the U.S. data for myocardial infarctions. *Compared to men, women—particularly those under age 55—were more than twice as likely to be mistakenly diagnosed; African Americans were four times more likely to be misdiagnosed.* The problem for women is some combination of discrimination and ignorance, the latter because presenting symptoms for females are more varied and less predictable than they are for men. For African Americans, one can only conclude that an unacceptable discrimination is at the heart of these problems. It is all too obvious that emergency services do not work as well for women and blacks as they do for men and whites.

CRITICAL CARE MEDICINE

Critical care is a new medical specialty. The first hospital coronary care units were introduced in the 1960s. The Society for Critical Care Medicine was founded in 1970, yet it was not until 1980 that physicians could be certified in critical care medicine. Initially, intensive care units (ICU) were organized to monitor vital signs in unstable patients, maintain airways, and provide mechanical ventilation for patients with reversible neurological conditions. Since its founding, the functions of the ICU have expanded considerably.

Like emergency intervention, critical care is concerned with the moment. Life hangs in the balance. Yet there are differences. The average emergency room stay is only three hours, and just one in twenty-five stay longer than a day; by contrast, a patient might stay for days in ICU.

Whereas a high proportion of emergency patients have life-threatening conditions, critical care medicine, by definition, is concerned exclusively with those patients who are at high risk of death. Yet for patients in ICU, the onset of risk may be gradual—deterioration from some chronic condition—as well as sudden. Finally, whereas emergency medicine begins within the community (e.g., programs to make available defibrillators and train personnel in their proper use), intensive care occurs at one site, the ICU. Purpose and goals aside, there is a direct effect between the emergency room and ICU: about one of every thirteen admissions to the former results in a transfer to the latter.

As always, our question is: What is the impact of critical care medicine on mortality? Does critical care save lives?

According to a Consensus Development Conference[22] on Critical Care Medicine, the answer is difficult to determine. Benefit is most evident for patients with acute reversible disease for whom the probability of survival without ICU is low. "When the risk of complication is high and the potential gain is large," wrote the CD panel in a statement of the obvious, "a decrease in mortality is likely." For other patient groups, the data are inconclusive. For cardiac care, the evidence is "equivocal, but the weight of clinical opinion is that ICU improves survival." For cardiogenic shock, "the weight of clinical opinion is that ICUs reduce mortality, though this conviction is supported only by uncontrolled or poorly controlled studies."

To their credit, the CD panel was careful to avoid unambiguous conclusions, rather relying on phrases such as "clinical opinion" and "uncontrolled studies." Even more worrisome, the panel pointed out that iatrogenic morbidity and mortality are "not infrequent, but not known with any precision."

"All this honesty is commendable," said Fran. "But it's not too reassuring."

Stated above are conclusions from 1983.[23] What has changed in the intervening years? The Society for Critical Care Medicine continues to publish a journal, founded in 1971. In the twenty-plus years since this CD, there has been much research on the efficacy of critical care, but little has changed from the conclusion presented therein.

The proposition that the ICU save lives surely has what is called "face validity," that is, it seems self-evident, and therefore not in need of formal proof. Each and every one of us knows of loved ones who have emerged, their lives intact, from critical care facilities. These stories are a form of knowledge that cannot and should not be ignored. Yet, such data cannot answer our question. Our best answer, such as it is, comes from a 2004 editorial from *Critical Care Medicine*: "It remains to be determined," wrote the editorialist, "what exactly it is in the delivery of critical care that confers a survival benefit."[24]

ALLIED SPECIALTIES

We briefly mention two related specialties, disaster medicine and battle-field medicine. Rather than treating the individual patient's emergency, disaster medicine is collective; it is a mass emergency: the earthquake, the flood, the terrorist attack—all of which cause problems of a different nature and far beyond anything seen in day-to-day medicine. Disasters may also be more common (and less dramatic) than generally thought. For example, a heat wave in Philadelphia from July 4 through July 14, 1993, caused a 26% increase in general mortality and a 98% increase in cardiovascular mortality—much of which was preventable.[25]

Far beyond the prehospital treatment of emergency medical service, disaster medicine begins at the cite, and must be ready to deal with power failures, water shortages and contamination, the decomposition of corpses, exposure to hazardous materials, evacuations, and panics. Disaster medicine has received considerable attention since the terrorist attack on the World Trade Center.[26] Most assessments claim that the United States is unprepared to face various disasters.

Battlefield medicine, which is nothing more than emergency medicine in the field, does save lives. In the Revolutionary War (1775–1783) an estimated 42% of all war wounds were lethal, a number that declined to 33% for the Civil War and only to 30% for World War II. In the current war (at this writing in 2005) in Iraq and Afghanistan, that figure has dropped to only 10%. "Though firepower has increased, lethality has decreased,"[27] claim the authors. This is undoubtedly true for the long course of history. Yet it seems to us that the low technology of this urban guerilla warfare, where the most dangerous weapons are so-called IEDs (improvised explosive devices), might have something to do with the higher rates of survival.

WHAT IF?

What if emergency medicine and its allied specialties disappeared?

As we have seen, an important (perhaps coequal) function of the emergency room, a function mandated by federal law, is to provide health care for uninsured and disadvantaged populations. In theory, it makes no sense whatever to have the same cite for the care of cardiac arrest and for safety net primary care—life and death on the one hand, routine on the other. Having these two disparate tasks leads to problems: overcrowding, deterioration of services, patient dumping, and to closing a significant number of emergency departments.

Even more, these problems with the safety net function interfere with the lifesaving function. An "onerous symptom" of this problem is that response times to real emergency calls continue to increase.[28] There is plenty wrong here, nothing short of scandalous for a country rich as ours. Yet our method in this book does not lead us down this particular path. We assess what is, not what ought to be. And in practice, at least in the United States, what we are stuck with is emergency care that also provides safety net care.

Thus, upon the disappearance of medicine, the quality of care for the disadvantaged would deteriorate considerably.

What about real emergency care? Would its absence lead to more deaths? Answering this question is problematic, given the understandable lack of controlled studies. Retrospective studies are similarly difficult to perform; one would need to compare the results of emergency care with some general or hypothetical population that did not receive such care.

Perhaps there is one good baseline comparison. In the United States, homicide rates have been declining since the 1960s. Yet during that same time aggravated assaults with firearms have tripled. What is the explanation for this apparent contradiction? It seem improbable that this decline is caused by a deterioration in shooters' aim. The difference seems to be the efficacy of the emergency system, probably in the efficiency of the "chain of survival." Mortality from gun assaults has fallen from 16% in 1964 to just 5% at the millennium.[29] Thus, we have indirect evidence of a substantial improvement in mortality from emergency medicine. Were medicine to vanish, it appears that more gunshot victims would die and, we presume, many others.

That which is distinctive about emergency medicine—its reliance on a "chain of survival" that occurs outside of, and prior to, the hospital—makes its disappearance particularly difficult to assess. Thus, our question is: How much of ER efficacy is due to what occurs prior to arrival at the hospital, prior to the care of physicians?

A 1975 study found that appropriate emergency care at the site and during ambulance transport accounted for a 62% reduction in coronary death and a 26% reduction for people over age 70. The authors concluded that:

Since prehospital cardiopulmonary resuscitation and emergency cardiac care have cheaply and effectively expedited and abbreviated hospitalization for acute myocardial infarction, and lowered community death rates from coronary artery disease, its adoption throughout the United States and the Western world seems justified.[30]

The "chain of survival" not only saves lives, but it is also not very expensive. There is widespread agreement that prehospital emergency care is cost-effective and "can contribute measurably to a reduction in heart disease mortality."[31] A Canadian assessment of prehospital treatment of heart attacks agreed, concluding that: (1) with minimal training, paramedics are capable of interpreting electrocardiograms and other diagnostics with equal skill to physicians; and (2) the earlier the treatment, the better the prognosis.

Thus, another piece of the puzzle: the "chain of survival" works, and works well, with paramedics who have little training, but with specific and situational diagnostic skills that match those of physicians. Given these findings, there is widespread agreement that "Communities should undertake all reasonable measures to optimize the provision of early CPR, early defibrillation, and prehospital ALS [advanced life support]."[32]

What are the policy implications of the success of the "chain of survival?" "Although direct comparisons are not feasible," claims a 2003 publication, "the immediate mortality benefit of EMS may be similar to that of bypass surgery."[33] This conclusion has two important implications for our book: the "chain of survival," which is community-based, holds great hope in keeping people alive; and bypass is less effective than generally touted in the popular media.

Saving lives is supposed to be the purview of the physician. The proposition that EMS personnel can prevent death is subversive; it undercuts the physician's supposedly unique authority. So is the corresponding proposition that members of the community (without advanced professional training) can save lives. Yet both propositions are true.

Consider the history of cardiopulmonary resuscitation. CPR was begun in the 1940s as a heroic open chest operation. By the 1960, it was demonstrated that closed chest massage was effective and could be performed in the ED. Initially, only physicians performed CPR, but nurses were soon taught the skill. During the 1970s, paramedics and then emergency medical technicians began performing CPR. In the 1980s, CPR was finally taught to the general public. Today, training in this potentially lifesaving skill is available through a wide variety of sites, including the World Wide Web.

The benefits of CPR are almost too good to be true. Sad to say, there is a problem, which is an issue we have seen time and again in this book: competence, or lack thereof. A 2005 study in *JAMA* found problems with out-of-hospital CPR. Paramedics did not deliver chest compressions half the time; when they did, most compressions were too shallow.[34] That was from a study of Sweden, Norway, and England. The same issue of *JAMA* presented a study of in-hospital CPR in Chicago. The findings? Compression was too slow in 28% of all cases, and too shallow in 37%. The quality of CPR "was inconsistent and often did not meet published guideline recommendations, even when performed by well-trained hospital staff."[35]

Does CPR quality make a life or death difference? One study found that patients who received "good" bystander CPR had significantly better hospital discharge rates than those who received poor CPR (23% vs. 6%). Another study showed a comparison of 16% to 4%.[36]

Our conclusion: CPR save lives. Properly done, CPR save more lives.

Real emergency medicine does save lives, and each life saved is of inestimable significance. Yet perhaps the great lesson of this chapter is that emergency medicine, which terminates in the ER, has its beginnings in the community. This "chain of survival," is not only cost effective, but also saves lives—perhaps more than, say, the much heralded cardiac bypass surgery. Indeed, the connection between hospital and community is one that needs strengthening, for the betterment of both personal and public health.

"The center cannot hold," wrote William Butler Yeats. "Mere anarchy is loosed upon the world."

With the disappearance of medicine, the center—the ER—would be gone. Some would die. But, interestingly, the edges would hold. The links in the "chain of survival" would not break. Some would also survive. Mere, but only mere, anarchy would be loosed upon the world.

5

PHARMACEUTICALS

in which we assess the impact of prescription drugs on mortality, and imagine a world without pharmaceuticals

The other day I was looking for something in my medicine cabinet. What I saw was a history of my various minor (knock wood!) afflictions over the past few years. There was a bottle of small red pills, marked: "take three times per day with food." What they were, and for what malady, I do not remember. I should have thrown them away. On either side of the suspect pills were bottles, one with two pills, the other with three. Both were antibiotics. More than likely, they never should have been prescribed in the first place; even so, I should have known better than to swallow them; yet once started, it's particularly stupid not to finish the prescription. Three wrongs cannot make a right.

Behind one of the antibiotics was a bottle of Vicodin.

It was prescribed a few years ago when I was having some dental pain. According to the *Physician's Desk Reference*, Vicodin is indicated for the "treatment of moderately severe pain." The pain wasn't very bad—not "moderately severe," whatever that means—so I never took any of the pills. A few months ago, Fran was having problems with her back. Her physician wrote a prescription for Vicodin. She refused to accept it.

It turns out that Vicodin is the most prescribed drug in the United States. In 2002, there were 139 million prescriptions written for "synthetic and semisynthetic narcotics." Of these, 81 million—with sales of

79

$1.5 billion—were for the generic category, hydrocodone, of which Vicodin is the best known brand. Use is increasing at breakneck speed. In 2002, there were 13.1 million people in the United States who had used Vicodin at least once. Just one year later, in 2003, the number was 15.7 million.

Semisynthetic narcotics have little to do with reducing mortality, our primary focus in this book. Yet there is little doubt that these drugs reduce pain, without doubt a laudable goal. "Narcotic pain medications are wonders of modern medicine for patients with serious pain who are under the care of physicians."[1] So said the Director of the Substance Abuse and Mental Health Administration (SAMHA) in 2004.

So far, so good.

Unfortunately, there is more. "When diverted from their legitimate use," continued the Director, "[these drugs] are highly addictive narcotics that the body perceives exactly as if the person were taking heroin."

I showed the quote to Fran first thing next morning. "They are hiding more than they are revealing."

"I can't talk before my first cup of coffee," she replied in a weak voice.

I was silent.

"What do they mean by 'legitimate,' Fran asked, ten minutes later, her large mug half empty.

"I don't know, but our government actually maintains that marijuana is the most commonly used illegitimate drug."

"What about underage drinking," she replied. "That's just as *illegitimate* and far more dangerous."

She was right, of course. Claiming that marijuana is more dangerous for kids than drinking is symptomatic of public health shortsightedness and stupid public policy.

At any rate, following marijuana in danger is the so-called nonmedical prescription use of natural (e.g., codeine) and semisynthetic narcotic pain relievers. About 30 million persons aged 12 or older (13% of the population) have used prescription pain relievers "nonmedically" in their lifetime. The number of drug abusers is increasing—rapidly. Those using prescription pain relievers nonmedically for the first time surged from 600,000 in 1990 to more than two million in 2001. Finally, about 1.5 million persons aged 12 or older were dependent on or abused prescription drug pain relievers in 2002.[2]

"What exactly do they mean by 'nonmedical?'"

"It's Clintonesque," I answered, thinking of our President's definition of "is!"

SAMHA defines "nonmedical" as the "use of prescription-type drugs not prescribed for the respondent by a physician or used only for the experience or feeling they caused."

For us, the definition, and therefore this entire discussion, is disingenuous.

First, SAMHA's notion of "experience" or "feeling" is vague and inadequate. If I take a pill to reduce pain, even one not prescribed for me, it will surely result in an "experience" that changes a "feeling." My pain will be ameliorated. In that case, I am using the pill exactly as it was intended, even though it was not intended for me. And what is the meaning of "only?" In addition to my change in "feeling," what else is supposed to happen? Other pills, legal and prescribed, are supposed to do nothing more—again, this notion of "only"—than cause changes in "experiences" or "feelings." Indeed, after semisynthetic narcotics, the entire category of "antidepressants"—pills designed only for the purpose of changing feelings— is next in prescription activity in the United States.

"Well, I feel better now," said Fran, putting down her empty coffee mug.

Second, no one makes Vicodin or any of the semisynthetic narcotics in his or her backyard laboratories. Every pill begins in a pharmaceutical laboratory and is transmitted to some person with a legal prescription. It is known that Vicodin is overprescribed, and inappropriately prescribed, by physicians.[3] Indeed, one can get the stuff—legally—without ever seeing a physician.

A few months ago, I was told that one could get these narcotics over the Internet. My first reaction was: how could this be possible without getting a prescription from a physician? I went online to one of many web sites, where I was directed to respond to a series of questions, being assured that a physician was carefully reviewing my answers. Were one to complete the process, Vicodin would arrive the following day by express post. Once I understood the process, I logged off with great offense. No harm done, I thought. But someone knows that I was shopping for the stuff. Someone is stealing my cookies! For I now routinely get e-mails, asking if I want to order Vicodin—or myriad other prescription drugs— each and all, I am assured, of the highest quality at the lowest price.

What all this means is that prescription drug abuse is not only a personal problem, but also an institutional one. Making and marketing drugs is what pharmaceutical companies do (we'll return to this issue at the chapter's conclusion); prescribing drugs is what physicians do; retailing them is what pharmacists do. For better or worse—and both outcomes are evident, though the latter is more frequent—each of these legal activities is tremendously profitable. Blaming the abuser is not inappropriate; blaming only the abuser is fallacious, as is not blaming the pharmaceutical industry and the medical industry. The neat distinction between "medical" and "nonmedical" is nothing more or less that an attempt to blame the victim—and only the victim—for his or her addiction.

No doubt: synthetic narcotics are a threat—a growing threat at that—to the public health. Unfortunately SAMHA's analysis lead us away from facing the problem, let alone finding a solution.

TRENDS

We need to throw out some numbers.

As Jonas Salk was putting the final touches on his vaccine in 1954, most drugs were sold over-the-counter (OTC). The best selling were Bufferin (Johnson & Johnson) and Geritol (Merck). By 2005, more than 100,000 preparations with 1,000 active ingredients were sold OTC. Annual sales exceeded $17 billion.[4]

Maybe there is something to be said for the 1950s nostalgia!

What about prescription drugs? At the midpoint of the twentieth century, the business was tiny. The two largest pharmaceutical companies at that time, Johnson & Johnson and Merck had, respectively, $204 and $1.5 million in prescription revenue. From 1960 to 1980, prescription sales were fairly static; from 1980 to 2000, they tripled. Since 1980, the pharmaceutical industry has consistently ranked as the most profitable in the United States In 2002, worldwide prescription sales were about $400 billion, half of which come from the United States.

In 1995, 2.12 billion prescriptions were filled in the United States; by 2002 that number had increased dramatically, almost 50%, to 3.14 billion, which comes to more than ten prescriptions per person! In 2002, about 10 million children took prescription medication for chronic conditions—that is, for three months or longer. During that same time period, retail sales more than doubled, from $72 billion to $182 billion, which is about $700 per capita. In 2001, prescription medicine expenses accounted for 18.5% of total health care spending in the United States.[5]

What is obvious and significant and central to this book is that in the brief period of seven years Americans are taking more drugs and spending more—much more—for them. As of 2003, more than 40% of all Americans—half of all women—take at least one prescription drug, and 17% take three or more.[6]

We are, it would seem, a drugged-up society.

The upsurging of prescription medications is the result of several factors: the growth of insurance coverage for drugs, the aggressive marketing of drugs by pharmaceutical companies, especially after a 1997 ruling that made it much easier for drug makers to advertise directly to the consumer, and clinical guidelines that recommend greater use of drugs to treat such conditions as high cholesterol, drug use for which tripled between 1995 and 2002.[7] Acute care is giving way to chronic or preventive care, for example, using drugs to manage high blood pressure. At the same time, disease treatment is being extended to therapy whose goal is to slow the aging process and promote well-being (e.g., drugs for what is called "male sexual dysfunction").

Instead of treating disease, as they once did, pharmaceutical companies have come to invent them! Consider heartburn as an instructive example. "The remedy used to be a glass of milk or an over-the-counter antacid" for symptomatic relief. Now heartburn is called "gastro-esophageal reflex disease (GERD)," a sign of serious esophageal disease, "which it is usually not." As a result of this "new" disease, by 2002 Prilosec was the third best-selling drug in the world, with sales exceeding $3 billion. Another example: the problems associated with menstruation were once a personal annoyance. Later they were called premenstrual syndrome (PMS) followed[8] by "premenstrual dysphoric disorder (PMDD), each redefinition requiring a more precise diagnosis and, of course, a different treatment regimen.

There is nothing new about creating new diseases solely for the purpose of treatment, as we will see in our discussion of estrogen replacement therapy. What we are witnessing is the worst of the medical model, which relentlessly seeks medical explanations and treatments for various and sundry behaviors—always, of course, with significant financial rewards.

RX

As we have said, semisynthetic narcotics (Vicodin and other brands) are the most commonly prescribed drug in the United States. Following that are the category of drugs for the treatment of depression, such as the brand Zoloft. Third in prescription activity are "statins," which are drugs that lower cholesterol (Lipitor and other brands). ACE inhibitors, for treatment of high blood pressure and chronic heart failure, are the fourth most commonly prescribed.

We've already considered semisynthetic narcotics; our discussion of antidepressants awaits the following chapter. Therefore, we turn our attention to...

Statins

Statins are a category of drug[9] that slow the body's ability to produce cholesterol and increase the liver's ability to remove low density lipids (LDLs), so-called bad cholesterol. We pose three questions: (1) do statins lower blood cholesterol? (2) do statins prevent heart attacks? (3) are statins effective in the treatment of heart disease?

First, there is widespread agreement that statins do lower blood cholesterol. According to the *Physician's Desk Reference: 2005*, there is a therapeutic response within weeks, with a maximum response in about four months. This effect is seen in male and females, and has been documented particularly in elderly populations. This result is dose dependent—the higher the dose, the greater the effect.

Second, are statins effective in primary prevention?

A 2004 article in the *New York Times* relates a "joke" among cardiologists that the benefits of statins are so great that they "should be added to the water supply." The article continues:

> Not only do statins greatly reduce cholesterol and lower mortality in people at risk for heart attacks, but some studies also suggest that they might help prevent or treat a wide range of ailments, including Alzheimer's disease, multiple sclerosis, bone fractures, some types of cancer, macular degeneration and glaucoma.[10]

Quite a list. Of all these claims, the most important is that statins prevent heart attacks, or other mortal events among those with high blood cholesterol. In other words, these people have a dangerous sign, presumably discovered from routine blood screening. They are thus at risk, but they do not have the disease, at least not in any way that can be detected. The prescription for this "problem" is said to be statins.

Three large clinical studies, all with acronym names,[11] have addressed the issue of primary prevention. The results from each were disappointing. There was a small reduction in heart attacks and strokes, but no change in overall mortality.

A meta-analysis of these and other studies, involving over 63,000 patients, concluded that "primary prevention with statins provides only small and clinically hardly relevant improvement of cardiovascular morbidity and mortality."[12] Another meta-analysis concluded that statins reduce the risk of stroke.[12] Yet one more meta-analysis showed that statins reduced heart attacks and strokes by 1.4% compared with the control. In other words, about 71 patients would need to be treated for 3 to 5 years to prevent one such event. There were no differences in mortality between those who took statins and those who took placebos. "Therefore, statins have not been shown to provide an overall health benefit in primary prevention trials."[14]

Thus, we arrive at two conclusions about statins and primary prevention: they have some small affect on morbidity (illness), but none on mortality.

There is one more issue. For any benefit, there also may be a corresponding risk.

Most experts claim that statins are remarkably safe, even over long periods of time; few side effects are noted. Yet one British study warns that "absolute safety of statins has not been demonstrated for patients at low risk of coronary heart disease."[15] And there have been problems. Bayer's Baycol was removed from the market in 2001 after reports that 31 people taking it had died from a rhamdomyolysis, a rare disorder involving muscle-tissue breakdown that leads to kidney failure. According to a 2004 article in *JAMA*, Bayer learned as early as 1999 that serious adverse reactions were associated with their drug. "To our knowledge," claim the *JAMA* authors, "these findings were not disseminated or published."[16]

These charges, serious indeed, perhaps criminal, were not reported in the mass media—as were allegations about another category of drugs, ACE inhibitors, which we discuss in a few pages.

"There's a multibillion industry ensuring that you hear all the good things [about statins]," said Dr. Bernice Golomb, principal investigator of a large federally financed study of the effects of statin on cognition, mental state, and other noncardiac processes.[17] But, she continued, "there is no corresponding interest group ensuring that you hear the other side." The widespread use of statins leads to other problems that are particularly significant for this book. "Most doctors give up on lifestyle changes because it takes an investment of time from both patient and physician," says one prominent physician. "It's easier to write a pre-scription for a statin."

"Maybe they shouldn't add statin to the water just quite yet," grum-bled Fran.

Alas, we have heard this magic pill rhetoric many times before, recently, for example, with hormone replacement therapy (see below). It was not true then. It's probably not true now.

Which is not to say that statins do no good.

Our third question is: Are statins effective in the treatment of heart disease?

Three major studies—again known by their acronyms[18]—have con-sidered this question. The answer is "yes."

The 4S research began in 1989. A five-year follow-up showed that statins reduced heart strokes and heart attacks by 36% and 43%, respec-tively. At that time, ethical considerations required that the placebo group be switched to statins. The ten-year follow-up still showed dra-matic improvement in the treatment group.

Do the other studies of secondary prevention show similar benefits? The answer is "yes." One meta-analysis, which included more than 47,000 subjects from five major outcome trials since 2002, concluded that statins reduced major coronary events by 27%, stroke by 18% and all-cause morality by 15%. Benefits accrued to both men and women, those with and without high blood pressure, diabetics and nondiabetics, and particularly for smokers.[19]

An editorial in the *New England Journal of Medicine* asserted that statins are effective in the treatment of stable coronary heart disease. Specifically, they "reduce the clinical consequences of atherosclerosis, including death from cardiovascular disease, nonfatal myocardial infarc-tion, nonfatal stroke, hospitalization for unstable angina pectoris and heart failure, as well as the need for [stenting]."[20]

To summarize: Statins are widely used in the United States. In 2002, more than 56 million prescriptions were written for Lipitor; as a group, statins were the third most prescribed drug. What can we conclude about their effectiveness? First, they do treat the sign. Blood cholesterol, particularly "bad (LDL) cholesterol" is reduced. One might therefore expect statins to be effective in the primary prevention of heart disease. Unfortunately and counterintuitively, treating the sign has little impact on dying from the disease. Statins are not effective in primary preven-tion. However, statins are effective in secondary prevention—that is, in preventing a recurrence of heart disease. In a book full of negative findings and criticism, it gives us great pleasure to review a carefully tested and efficacious treatment that undoubtedly saves lives.

ACE INHIBITORS

Angiotensin converting enzyme (ACE) inhibitors[21] are a category of drug that relax blood vessels and thereby lower blood pressure; this same action allows the heart to work less hard and therefore ACE inhibitors are a common treatment for congestive heart failure.

As with statins, we pose three questions: (1) Do they lower blood pressure? (2) Are they effective in primary prevention; that is, do ACE inhibitors prevent first-time heart attacks (fatal or nonfatal) in patients with high blood pressure? (3) Are they effective secondary prevention, that is, in the treatment of heart conditions?

First, it is evident that ACE inhibitors lower blood pressure. According to the *Physician's Desk Reference*, within two weeks, they lower systolic and diastolic pressure, respectively, by 2–10 mm and 4–6mm mercury.

Second, unfortunately, there is no evidence that ACE inhibitors are effective in primary prevention of congestive heart failure. In 2003, A meta-analysis of 42 clinical trials involving almost 200,000 patients concluded that they had little effect. Moreover, and to the surprise of all, low dose diuretics were more effective than ACE inhibitors in the prevention of cardiovascular morbidity or mortality. "Clinical practice and treatment should reflect this evidence," concluded the authors.[22] Unfortunately, and once again counterintuitively, treating the sign does not necessarily prevent the disease. The principal author of one major clinical trial said: "We find out now that we've wasted a lot of money. In addition, [the current practice] has probably caused harm to patients."[23]

"How embarrassing," I commented.

"It's more than embarrassing. It's malpractice," countered Fran.

There is a lesson here. In 1982, diuretics accounted for 56% of prescriptions written for blood pressure; ten years later, after ACE inhibitors were marketed, they accounted for 27%. A list of the best-selling drugs among senior citizens shows three ACE inhibitors, but no diuretics. We have replaced the inexpensive drug with an expensive one.

Third, ACE inhibitors do have a limited effect in reducing the risk of heart failure and death from strokes. The HOPE study found that the treated group suffered fewer heart failures (9% compared to the 11.5%

for the placebo), fewer deaths from diabetes (6.4% compared with 7.6%), and fewer deaths from all causes (10.4% to 12.2%).[24] A meta-evaluation of five major studies involving more than 12,000 patients found similar results. Treatment led to fewer heart failures (13.7% to 18.9%) and fewer deaths from any cause (23% to 26.8%).[25]

For other conditions of the heart, ACE inhibitors do not seem to be effective. In the PEACE Trial, 21.9% of the treatment group, compared with 22.5% of the placebo group, died within five years. "There is no evidence that the addition of ACE inhibitors," wrote the authors, "provides further benefit in terms of death from cardiovascular disease, myocardial infarction, or coronary revascularization."[26] A Japanese study showed similar negative results. About 2,000 patients who had suffered acute myocardial infarctions were either treated with ACE inhibitors or placebos. Both groups suffered an annual rate of fatal or nonfatal cardiac events of 32%.[27]

What can we conclude about ACE inhibitors? As with statins, they do treat the sign. Blood pressure is reduced. As with statins, we would expect them to be effective in primary prevention; as with statins, they are not. An innovative statistical analysis found that preventing one cardiac event (fatal or nonfatal) would require treating 1,653 persons with ACE inhibitors, compared to 1,181 with statins.

ACE inhibitors are effective, though not as dramatically as statins, in the secondary prevention of heart disease. To avoid one recurrent cardiac event would require treating 69 people with ACE inhibitors compared to 53 people with statins. Thus, ACE inhibitors can and do save lives, though not as efficiently as statins. And this, ACE inhibitors work only slightly better than aspirin—for which 93 people must be treated to avoid a cardiac event![28] Two conclusions are clear. Compared to ACE inhibitors, common diuretics work better for primary prevention; aspirin works almost as well for secondary prevention.

TWO MORALITY TALES

Problems notwithstanding, ACE inhibitors, and especially statins, have saved lives. Our readers, having gotten this far in this book, surely welcomed the generally good news. And rightly so. Nonetheless, our task is to investigate (and, as we said in chapter 1, to debunk), not to feel good. With that in mind, we turn our attention to two cases since the turn of the millennium. Both of these—hormone replacement therapy for treatment of menopausal symptoms, and so-called Cox-2 inhibitors, which are pain relievers—are medical morality tales from which we may learn many important lessons.

Hormone Replacement Therapy

We would like to think that the development of new drugs follows a prudent and rational procedure: that research protocols are carefully designed and evaluated, and that decisions about dosage and use are evidence-based, so that ultimately such drugs are both safe and effective.

Unfortunately, when Fran studied the estrogen replacement controversy,[29] she found something very different.

This particular telling of the story begins in the early 1960s, when the medical profession hailed estrogens as the fountain of youth and beauty, and as the elixir of femininity and sexuality. Prominent gynecologists "discovered" that menopause was a deficiency disease, just like diabetes. And just like diabetes, it had a cure. A bold promise was made that so-called estrogen replacement therapy (ERT) would let women avoid menopause entirely and keep them "feminine forever," the title of a popular and widely quoted book by gynecologist Robert Wilson.

Wilson described menopause as "living decay," but said that estrogens could "save women from being condemned to witness the death of their womanhood." He listed 26 physiological and psychological symptoms that the "youth pill" could avert, and, in an article in the *Journal of the American Geriatrics Society*, advocated that women be given estrogens from "puberty to grave."

Another gynecologist promoted estrogens as "an energizer, tranquilizer and antidepressant that stimulates mental capacity, memory, and concentration, restores the zest for living, and gives a youthful appearance." Yet another wrote that without estrogen "a women comes as close as she can to being a man." They "live in a world of intersex. Having outlived their ovaries, they have outlived their usefulness as human beings."

What an amazing collection of health claims, none backed by research, but all surrounded by a large dose of misogyny!

As it turned out, estrogens are effective in controlling menopausal hot flashes. Otherwise, each and every one of these medical claims proved to be false.

Nonetheless, between 1963 and 1975, dollar sales for prescription estrogen replacements quadrupled. As one Harvard researcher noted:

"Few medical interventions have had as widespread application as exogenous estrogen treatment in postmenopausal women." By 1975, with prescriptions at an all time high of 30 million, estrogens had become the fifth most widely prescribed drug in the United States. Sales of estrogens amounted to $85 million, of which the brand, Premarin, were $70 million.

Then came the discovery in 1975 that ERT increased by four to twenty times the likelihood of endometrial cancer, followed by research that linked ERT to increase the risk of heart attacks, artery disease, blood clots, and diabetes. No one should have been surprised, for the link between estrogens and various diseases, especially cancer, was well known. "Another human experiment has been set up in recent years by the widespread administration of estrogens to postmenopausal women," wrote a researcher four decades earlier, in 1947, who then criticized the practice as "promiscuous."

Because of the cancer scare, prescriptions for estrogens had by 1979 declined dramatically to 16 million. Even so, the Food and Drug Administration (FDA) concluded that estrogens were still "grossly overused." Fran's analysis of 1979 prescriptions revealed that 31% were still written for such vague diagnostic categories as "symptoms of senility," "special conditions without sickness," and "mental problems"—all in explicit violation of FDA specifications.

That should have been the end of the story. Menopause had been inappropriately medicalized. A disease had been invented for which a treatment, estrogen, was a cure. The idea was nonsense, though very profitable nonsense. Menopause is a natural occurrence—not a malady—for all healthy women. The problematic symptoms of menopause can be ameliorated without putting women at risk of cancer and other deadly diseases.

Alas, that was not the end of the story. Throughout the 1980s and 1990s, postmenopausal women took estrogen along with progestin, a combination that purportedly offered the benefits of the old ERT, for maladies ranging from hot flashes to osteoporosis, as well as protection from heart disease and breast cancer. Risks from this so-called hormone replacement therapy (HRT) were denied or minimized. A survey conducted in 1995 showed that about 38% of women aged 50 to 75 were using HRT. At the turn of millennium, some 55 million postmenopausal women were on HRT.[30]

Yet there were problems. Several studies done in the late 1990s found that many of the expected benefits never materialized; even worse,

HRT raised the risk of the very diseases—breast cancer and heart disease—that it was purported to prevent.[31] In 2002 and 2003, the Women's Health Initiative demonstrated that HRT actually increased the risk of both breast cancer and cardiovascular disease and breast cancer[32] and as well increased the risk of Alzheimer's Disease—though HRT had been thought to increase cognitive activity.[33]

"*Deja vu*, all over again," muttered Fran, quoting another president.

For all these problems, the increased risks were termed "small." What "small" means is that HRT's use was responsible for 3,500 cardiac disease events, 2,000 breast cancers, 4,000 strokes, and 5,000 cases of pulmonary embolism per annum. For those women who are part of these numbers, they are, of course, life-changing events. Yet, despite the way it might sound, this is indeed a small fraction of the total population of users. However, any risk, no matter the size, is not worth taking if there is no counterbalancing benefit. As it turns out, the purported benefits of HRT never materialized. The lead author of the 2003 WHI study put it well: "Do you want to take an intervention... that will reduce hot flashes 90 percent, probably at the cost of having a one in 25 chance of an abnormal mammogram?"[34]

By 2003, the number of women using HRT had declined by 50%. Even so, Wyeth Pharmaceuticals, which produces Prempro, the most popular brand of HRT, projected profits of about $1.5 billion for 2004.

For us, the story of ERT, and then the almost repeat story of HRT, is frustrating. Numerous clinical studies show that there is little or nothing to be gained from estrogen treatments, and much to be lost. Yet a confluence of interests—pharmaceutical companies pushing drugs for diseases that they invented, professional imperialism, and the cultural stereotyping of aging women—has too much momentum to stop. This is not an example of bad science so much as an example of inappropriate and even dangerous medical practice. And this: We should be more than a bit suspicious of claims about pills that produce fountains of youth or any other miracle.

COX-2 Inhibitors

We begin our story long after the beginning.

In September, 2004, the National Institutes of Health (NIH) announced that it had halted a clinical trial of Vioxx because it caused a twofold increase in "major fatal and nonfatal cardiovascular events."[35] In November of the same year, the FDA claimed that Vioxx might have contributed to an estimated 27,785 fatal and nonfatal heart attacks from 1999 through 2003. A month later, the NIH announced that there were problems in a study with a closely related drug, Celebrex. This time a 2.5 fold increase in major heart problems was observed.

In response, Merck withdrew Vioxx from the marketplace; Pfizer, maker of Celebrex, did not. At that time, annual sales of Vioxx were $2.5 billion; Celebrex, the seventh most prescribed drug in the United States (21 million prescriptions in 2003), had sales of $3.3 billion per annum.[36]

The story actually began in the 1980s, when scientists studying cancer discovered a naturally occurring substance (COX-2) that contributed to inflamation and cell proliferation. In the late 1990s, its antagonists (COX-2 inhibitors) were developed into designer drugs called nonsteroidal anti-inflammatory drugs of which the best know were Vioxx and Celebrex (Aleve and Advil are over-the-counter versions). These drugs purported to relieve pain and inflammation without causing—as did aspirin—an estimated 16,500 deaths from stomach ulcers and bleeding; it was also believed that they inhibited cell proliferation, thereby being a treatment for cancer.

COX-2 inhibitors were declared another miracle drug. In 2002, the CEO of Pfizer rhapsodized over Celebrex: "Millions of people who were once crippled with arthritis can now work, walk, garden, and do all the little things that make life worthwhile."[37]

Amidst the explosion of sales and use, especially for the relief of pain from arthritis and other chronic conditions, there were rumblings of problems. In 2001, a team of researchers led by Eric Topol[38] published a meta-analysis in *JAMA* showing that Vioxx use increased the risk of heart attacks fivefold.[39] In response, Merck conducted its own study which found a much smaller risk.

In December 2004, a meta-analysis of 18 clinical trials of Vioxx was published in the highly respected British journal, *Lancet*. It found that patients given Vioxx had 2.3 times the risk of heart attacks compared with those given placebos or other medications, and that this relationship was known as early as the year 2000. "Our findings," write the researchers, "indicate that [Vioxx] should have been withdrawn several years earlier."[40]

When did Merck and Pfizer find out about their COX-2 problems? According to the *Wall Street Journal*, internal Merck e-mails reveal that the company knew the potential risks of their best-selling drug as early as the year 2000. Merck's marketing literature included documents for its sales representatives which discussed how to respond to questions about Vioxx.

It was labelled "Dodge Ball Vioxx!"[41]

And Pfizer? In October 2004, the company asserted that it had no studies prior to that year which indicated problems with Celebrex. Alas, in February 2005, the company admitted that a 1999 trial showed a dramatic increase in cardiovascular problems. The study was never published; it was submitted to the FDA in 2001, four months after a major review of Vioxx and Celebrex.[42]

In a 2004 *Lancet* editorial, Richard Horton called Vioxx a "public health catastrophe" and accused Merck and the FDA of "ruthless, short-sighted and irresponsible self-interest."[43] He especially criticized the FDA for failing to act as early as 2001, and called for a complete restructuring of that agency. Strong words, indeed. In an interview, Eric Topol said that he had "never read a more powerful editorial in a medical journal."[44]

In a "Perspective" of the *New England Journal of Medicine*, Topol concluded:

> It is clear to me that Merck's commercial interest in [Vioxx] sales exceeded its concern about the drugs potential cardiovascular toxicity. Had the company not valued sales over safety, a suitable trial could have been initiated rapidly at a fraction of the cost of Merck's direct-to-consumer advertising campaign.[45]

Writing from the "editorial desk" (which clearly gives the writer more authority than a "letter to the editor") of the *New York Times*, Topol estimated that COX-2 inhibitors were responsible for tens of thousands of heart attacks or strokes per annum. "Good riddance to a bad drug," he concluded, calling the entire story of COX-2 inhibitors "a debacle."[46]

That should have been the end of the story. Not so. On February 18, 2005, an advisory panel for the FDA voted unanimously that Vioxx and Celebrex can lead to serious heart problems. Most of the panel also recommended warning labels that detailed the drug's danger and also a ban on consumer advertising. The panel then voted 31–1 that Pfizer should be allowed to continue selling Celebrex, and 17–15 that Merck could sell Vioxx.[47]

"At least the pharmaceutical lawyers must be happy," I said. "The panel's endorsement of both drugs will definitely help Merck and Pfizer fend off the hundreds of lawsuits already filed by patients and their survivors."

The panel's chairman, trying to put the whole debacle in perspective, made the unfortunate comment: "It would be a brave man or woman [physician] who started a patient with a clear history of heart disease on these drugs."[48]

"That's not brave," complained Fran. "It's either incompetent or negligent.!"

What are the lessons of COX-2 Inhibitors for our book?

We live in a hypermodern society. Everything happens at breakneck speed. Vioxx, the first of the COX-2 inhibitors, was approved for marketing in 1999. The pharmaceutical companies made billions of dollars in profits, in part by inappropriate (though legal) direct advertising. Olympic gold medalists Dorothy Hamill and Bruce Jenner did television endorsements for Vioxx. Three Dog Night sang, "Celebrate," to sell Celebrex. Five years later it was all over. Commentators used the label "debacle," "folly," and other synonyms to summarize what happened.

Such judgments miss the point.

If it is true that Merck, Pfizer, and other pharmaceutical companies knew the truth about cardiovascular dangers, then they are fully culpable in tens of thousands of deaths.

"That's murder," whispered Fran.

But what about pain relief? What about allowing people to "work, walk, garden, and do all the little things that make life worthwhile?" We repeat two scientific findings: first, COX-2 inhibitors really do hospitalize and even kill people; second, amazingly, they are no better at relieving pain than over-the-counter medications, a finding which was published a full year before the Pfizer CEO's rhapsody.[49]

THE AMERICAN PHARMACY

Remember the millennial article in the *New England Journal* from the first page of this book. "Medicine is one of the few spheres of human activity," wrote the *Journal's* editors, "in which the purposes are unambiguously altruistic." It goes without saying that this statement is not true, or at best a caricature of the truth. Like all other major social institutions, medicine has an economic base—and is typified by the pursuit of self-interest. And there is nothing wrong with that. Yet there are institutional controls which are supposed to place checks and balances on the pecuniary aspects of medicine.

For the drugs reviewed in this chapter—from best-selling Vicodin to Vioxx—these institutional restraints were either not applied or not enforced with vigor. In each case, some combination of pharmaceutical companies, governmental regulatory agencies, and physicians acted, and in some cases continue to act, irresponsibly— even criminally.

Even so, we might hold to the notion that the system of drug development and distribution does great good in our world. Were it only so!

Marcia Angell, former editor-in-chief of the *New England Journal of Medicine*, wrote of two myths that enshroud the pharmaceutical industry: First, it spends huge amounts of capital on the development of new drugs (which justifies the high prices for their products); and second that in so doing, it produces a significant number of new drugs.

What about the vaunted research and development (R&D)? In 2002, according to Angell, the industry spent $31 billion (14% of its sales) on R&D, compared to its profits, which were $36 billion (17%). More startling is that they spent $67 billion (31%)—almost double their R&D budgets—on "marketing and administration." The industry claims that it spends $802 million on the development of each new drug, a cost that justifies high retail prices. Angell recalculated the cost at about $100 million. In all, and by any measure, the industry invests precious little in R&D, and therefore—despite its public presentation—is not an innovative industry.

Second, what do we get for that money? Very little, it would seem. Most new drugs are so-called me-too, meaning that they are chemical variations of existing drugs. For example, with its patent for Prozac about to lapse, Eli Lilly became quite creative. It renamed Prozac to Sarafem, colored it pink, and got FDA approval to market it for "premenstrual disphoric disorder" (PMDD). "Same drug, same dose, but priced three and a half times higher than generic Prozac."[50] Of the 78 drugs approved by the FDA in 2002, only 17 contained new ingredients, and only seven were classified by the FDA as improvements over existing drugs.

All that capital, all that effort: all for seven really new drugs!

Surely this is further evidence of the lack of innovation in the big drug companies.

There is a related problem. The pharmaceutical industry has compromised the scientific process that supposedly underlies their existence. And we, the people, or at least our government, have let them do it! The very clinical trials which are crucial in establishing a new drug's efficacy are designed, carried out, and interpreted not by independent investigators, but by the very drug companies that have an enormous vested interest in the outcomes.

The government agency that is supposed to regulate the industry is the FDA. It has not done its job, especially in recent years. One problem is that the agency is under undue influence from the very industry it regulates. Since 1992, drug companies have paid "user fees" to the FDA. In 2002, this amounted to $576,000 per new drug application, for a total of $260 million. Sad to say, that money, now an integral part of the FDA budget, buys considerable influence. Add to that the practice of using outside experts to help the FDA reach its decisions. At 92% of these meetings in the year 2000, one expert had a financial conflict of interest, and at 55% of the meetings, at least half the members had a conflict of interest.[51] This does not mean that consultants are dishonest, but it does raise considerable suspicion.

There are also inevitable organizational problems for the FDA. Indeed, the mission of the FDA contains inherent contradictions that lead to inevitable dissonance. "It is unreasonable," wrote the editors of *JAMA*, "to expect the same agency that was responsible for approval of drug licensing and labeling would also be committed to actively seek evidence to prove itself wrong." What is needed, the editors continued, is for Congress to establish an "independent drug safety board" to track the safety of drugs and medical devices after they are approved for use. Above all, "this agency must be completely independent of influence from the pharmaceutical industry, biotechnology firms, and medical device manufacturers."[52]

If the connections between the companies and their regulators are suspicious, so are the ties between the industry and physicians. The pharmaceutical industry employs about 88,000 sales representatives, which comes to about one for every five physicians. It is their job to "educate" physicians on the purported benefits of particular drugs. To put it bluntly, these company employees bribe physicians with gifts large and small. The AMA instructs physicians not to take gifts, and in 2002, the industry adopted a "voluntary" code of conduct to "discourage" expensive gifts. Three years later, according to the FDA's Acting Director Commissioner for Operations, nothing had changed; sales representatives were still "showering" physicians with gifts.[53]

All evidence suggests that physicians listen closely to these sales representatives, who have no advanced degrees in the biomedical sciences. For the physician to fall under such influence is tantamount to inappropriately and dangerously ceding his or her hard-won expertise. "To rely on drug companies for unbiased evaluation of their products makes about as much sense as relying on beer companies to teach us about alcoholism." So wrote commented Angell, when she was still editor of the *New England Journal of Medicine.*

WHAT IF?

If medicine were to disappear, so would the pharmaceutical industry. What would result?

We have discovered that the huge and vaunted pharmaceutical industry accomplishes less—in terms of saving lives—than one might expect. Seven new drugs in 2002 is hardly a great record. But, let us review the efficacy of the best-selling drugs. Semisynthetic narcotics save no lives. They do alleviate pain, no small achievement, but this accomplishment must be balanced against their widespread misuse. The routine use, and even legitimate prescription of, Vicodin is a national scandal. As a nation, we take far too many narcotics, and it should come as no surprise that many of us, more every year, are addicted.

We will discuss antidepressants, the next most often prescribed category of drugs, in the following chapter. Suffice to say, they don't work very well, let alone save lives.

Statins, in third place, are ineffective in the prevention of cardiovascular problems, but they are effective in treating recurrent disease—an accomplishment we dare not overlook. Next in prescription activity are ACE inhibitors, which, surprisingly (scandalously!) work no better than diuretics.

Neither estrogens or COX-2 inhibitors are miracle drugs. The former do not accomplish much and in fact cause considerable morbidity and some mortality. The latter are no more effective in relieving pain than less powerful substances; what they do is kill people.

Many of the presumed diseases treated by prescription drugs are not pathological, but rather clusters of symptoms, the origins of which are either social, psychological, or from the natural process of aging—or most likely, a combination of all three. If medicine were to disappear, so would most cases of PMDD, ED, and other invented alphabet soup conditions.

Widespread use of drugs has inverted the entire diagnostic system. For example, shortness of breath or chest pain are symptoms; elevated cholesterol is the sign. In the medical model, the latter takes precedence over the former, especially since the sign itself, even in the absence of the symptom, becomes a flag that indicates some cardiovascular pathology.

Here is the rub. In the absence of any symptom or even in the absence of any pathology, the sign is taken to predict the future onset of pathology. The sign itself must be further explored with expensive tests and treated with powerful and expensive drugs, perhaps over long periods of time. That the logic doesn't work too well was demonstrated in this chapter, where the sign, detected in routine exam, may be a poor predictor of disease, especially mortal disease.

The way around that problem is to call the sign itself the disease, a phenomenon which is professionally and financially advantageous, but which does not demonstrably improve the health of the American people.

Can we find drugs that work well and save lives? Of course. Their loss would be significant, but, perhaps, not as great as might be imagined.

We can also find ones—best-selling ones—that are safe for most people, but from time to time take lives. Remember from chapter I that adverse reactions to correctly prescribed drugs kill an estimated 106,000 hospitalized patients per year, which is, amazingly, the fifth leading cause of death, just ahead of "accidents" (98,000 in 1999).

What if prescription drugs disappeared? Recall that we are talking about just a handful of new drugs per year. Even so, lives would surely be lost. But some would also be saved. In the research literature there is no calculation of the presumed good balanced against the possible harm. The very act of asking such a question—which is precisely what we are doing—is subversive, for it implies that a negative answer is possible. From the evidence reviewed herein, it appears that were drugs to disappear, mortality would not much be affected.

The findings from this chapter are a disappointment to us and should be for all readers. The policy recommendations from this discussion will be developed in our concluding chapter. Considering the massive and constantly growing expenditure, the immense hype, and the vaunted expectations, it appears that little is accomplished in the reduction of mortality. Surely a society so interested in its health can and should do better.

6

MENTAL ILLNESS

*in which we assess the concept and treatment of mental
health, and imagine a world without psychiatry*

At the turn of the millennium, Americans had their televisions
tuned to the critically acclaimed series, *The Sopranos*. The protagonist,
Tony, was a Mafia boss who on occasion murdered people—with considerable violence and little remorse. He had normal (which is to say problematic) relations with his teenage children. He loved his wife, though
regularly cheated on her. He also—here the plot thickened—was being
treated by a psychoanalyst.

What was Tony's problem? Was he a psychopathic personality or
merely narcissistic? Perhaps "depression" was a more appropriate diagnosis. Were his fainting episodes an expression of panic disorder? His psychiatrist treated him with psychotherapy, and also with Prozac, which
abated his panic attacks but not the depression. She then prescribed
lithium, for a "kick start," followed by higher doses of Prozac. His condition worsened; his diagnosis remained unclear.

The closest (and perhaps wisest) observer of Tony's condition was
his wife, Carmela. In one episode, she offered him a more than skeptical diagnosis: "I can't tell if you're just old-fashioned, paranoid, or a
fuckin' asshole."[1]

Carmela's conundrum captures this chapter's problems. How
common is mental illness? How is it defined—that is, are there clear

demarcations between nasty or nonnormative behavior as opposed to behaviors that result from something that we would call "an illness?" Should such conditions be treated by psychiatrists, and if so, with what modality? And finally: How effective are standard treatments?

PREVALENCE

Tony Soprano was not alone. Many people are afflicted with what are defined as serious emotional or mental problems.[2] According to the National Institute of Mental Health (NIMH), about one in five adults—some 45 million people—suffer from a diagnosable mental disorder in any given year. Three of the leading ten causes of disability (major depression, bipolar disorder, and schizophrenia) are mental disorders. The most serious of these problem may lead to suicide. In the year 2000, about 29,000 Americans took their own lives. More than 90% of them suffered from a diagnosable mental disorder. Men commit suicide four times more often than women, however women attempt suicide 2–3 times as often as men.[3]

How accurate are these numbers? Establishing just how many people suffer from mental illness—that is, national estimates of prevalence—is problematic. There are two possible sources of information: First, we can collect data from treatment sites, such as visits to doctors' offices, pharmaceutical prescriptions filled, or even hospital admissions; most of the information we consider subsequently in this chapter is from these sources.

Second, we can collect data from typical citizens regarding their possible mental problems.[4] The National Comorbidity Survey did just that, administering a structured psychiatric interview to a random sample of 8,000 Americans from 1990 to 1992. The findings: 30% of working adults had experienced a diagnosable mental illness in the previous year (18% if substance abuse is not counted). Almost half (48%) had experienced a diagnosable mental illness in their lifetime (21% without substance abuse). The most common illnesses were major depression and alcohol abuse, reported by 10% and 7%, respectively. Only 0.7% reported ever having a psychotic illness.[5]

Mental illness is not randomly distributed in the population. Men consistently display higher rates of substance abuse and "chronic maladaptive" personality traits, such as gambling or antisocial behaviors; more common among women are anxiety disorders and depression.

"Gender roles," Fran said. So much of who we are, male and female, comes from gender roles."

"And don't forget social class," I added, for we knew that as socioeconomic status increases, diagnosable mental illness and psychological distress decrease."[6]

"Money doesn't always help," Fran concluded, "but it almost never hurts."

PSYCHIATRISTS

In previous chapters, we have considered the impact of some particular medical specialty on mortality. This chapter is different. For the most part, psychiatrists do not deal with life or death issues. Their disappearance would have little effect on mortality. Why, then, should we devote a chapter to psychiatry and mental illness?

The answer is twofold. First, however defined and with whatever issues of validity, mental illness is a very large problem in the United States; and second, there are, in the United States, 16.5 psychiatrists per 100,000 population, the most of any country in the world.[7] At the new millennium, psychiatry was the fourth largest medical specialty in the United States.[8] The best estimate of the number of active clinically trained practicing psychiatrists in the private sector is 45,000,[9] only a small proportion of whom (3–6%) restrict themselves to inpatient practice. The specialty has grown rapidly (from 1970 to 2002, the number of psychiatrists increased by 86%), though recent evidence shows a downward reversal of that trend.[10]

A comparison of surveys of psychiatrists done in 1989 and 1996 shows two important demographic trends: the proportion of women is increased rapidly, from 19% to 25%; and those over age 55 increased from 32% to 38%. Indeed there has been a 40% decline in the percent of U.S. medical school graduates entering first year residencies in psychiatry. According to the 1996 survey, about half of all treatments were done in the psychiatrist's offices; mood disorders accounted for the greatest proportion of caseloads (36%), followed by patients with anxiety disorders (14%) and schizophrenia and other psychotic disorders (13%).[11]

Until a few decades ago, the psychiatrist treated the patient with "talk therapy." Today the treatment is drugs. A survey of psychiatrists, conducted in 1997, showed that 89% of all patients received at least one psychotherapeutic medication; 14% received four or more medications. The most commonly prescribed drugs were antidepressants (62% of all patients), followed by antianxiety agents (32%) and antipsychotic agents (27%).[12]

DSM

Our evaluation of psychiatry—be it therapy with talk or drugs—is made difficult by the very issue that vexes the practice. That is, what psychiatrists do has never really fit into the medical model. The problem is that while there are surely symptoms of mental illness, there are in most cases no signs. We routinely refer to being "depressed" (which is a distressingly loose set of symptoms) as "clinical depression," which is then explained as a biochemical imbalance. Yet, at least to date, blood, urine, and other body fluids yield no reliable indicator of a problem—for example, that above or below a certain metric the patient suffers from some disease, say something called "depression."[13]

Is so-called mental illness really an illness?[14]

A good starting place is to examine the American Psychological Association's (APA) position on this issue. As it happens, this organization publishes (and gives its official imprimatur) to an inclusive list, in the form of a classification, of mental illnesses. The first edition of the *Diagnostic and Statistical Manual* (*DSM*) was published in 1952. That edition and the second one took a psychodynamic approach to mental illness in which the cause of problems was generally attributed to the environment. There were no sharp distinction between normal and abnormal, between those who were mentally ill and those who were not. Everyone had various and sundry difficulties; people with more severe problems had more trouble functioning, and thus were in need of treatment. Considerable effort was made to distinguish between psychosis and neurosis, the former involving a complete break with reality, the latter characterized by anxiety and depression.

All that changed with the publication in 1980 of *DSM-III*. The psychodynamic model was abandoned in favor of a medical model, which introduced—as should be clear from our discussion in chapter 1—a clear distinction between the normal and the abnormal. Either one was mentally ill, in which case a specific and unique diagnosis was necessary, or one was not mentally ill. "Each of the mental disorders," according to the editors

is conceptualized as a clinically significant behavioral or psychological syndrome...associated with either a painful symptom (distress) or impairment in one or more areas of functioning (disability)....There is behavioral, psychological, or biological dysfunction...the disturbance is not only in the relationship between the individual and society.[15]

The third edition gave considerable attention, previously absent, to the logic and actual process of diagnosis. Some categories were expanded. For example, anxiety neurosis became a number of discreet disorders, including social phobia, generalized anxiety disorder, panic disorder, posttraumatic stress disorder (PSTD), and obsessive-compulsive disorder. At the same time, the diagnosis of "neurosis" was eliminated, the word itself disappearing entirely from the newer volumes. *DSM-IV*, published in 1996, continued to emphasize differential diagnosis, as did *DSM-IV-TR* (text revision), published in 2000.[16] For example, the one category for "disorders of sleep" was replaced by 15 different categories, ranging from "primary insomnia" to "breathing-related sleep difficulties."

Thus, over time, *DSM-IV* became, in the words of its editors, a detailed "classification of mental disorders that was developed for use in clinical, educational and research settings."[17] Yet even as it became a standard reference, its wise authors recognized that they are dealing with muddy foundational concepts.[18]

Some scholars, psychiatrists among them, rejected the very notion that emotional problems are illnesses. Every normal person has various complaints, some much worse and more serious than others. But to call "complaints about the body illnesses, despite the objective evidence of illness," wrote psychiatrist and critic Thomas Szasz, "is a violation of elementary rules of logic, an offense against scientific medicine, and an act of medical hubris." Indeed paging through the *DSM* is an odd exercise, for it lists without in great detail traditional and serious personality traits along with problems most of us would consider less serious, for example, ones related to caffeine intake. "The primary function and goals of the *DSM*," contends Szasz, "is to lend credibility to the claim that certain (mis)behaviors are mental disorders and that such disorders are mental diseases. Thus, pathological gambling enjoys the same status as myocardial infarction."[19]

Because of the prominence of the *DSM*, and because of its scientific and existential claims, we can examine the *DSM* itself as a proxy for understanding what is meant by the notion of mental illness. The first edition of the *DSM* was 128 pages in length and enumerated 106 diagnoses. Each edition has grown. The fourth edition (text revised) now has 943 pages and enumerates 365 diagnoses. Thus, in five decades the number of specific diagnoses has tripled.

One psychiatrist critic offered two hypotheses to explain the growth of the *DSM*: that with advances in medical science, we can now "identify mental illnesses that were there all along, but went unrecognized" because of our "primitive knowledge"; alternatively, "we are witnessing the expansion of mental health professions, which label as mental disorders human behaviors that only four decades ago were considered either medical disorders or routine difficulties of ordinary life." As we might expect, the writer chose the latter hypothesis, concluding that "there is far more pseudoscience than real science in the *DSMs*."[20]

Good science or not, the *Manual* and its categories of illness have real consequences. First, it allows the patient to assume what more than a half century ago sociologist Talcott Parsons called the "sick role." The sick person (1) is exempt from normal responsibilities; (2) is not responsible for his or her illness; (3) must try to become well; and (4) therefore must seek, and, most importantly, take the advice of professional help. Consider alcoholism. A bad drinking problem has become a disease called "alcohol use disorder," be it, according to *DSM-IV-TR*, "alcohol dependence" (303.90) or "alcohol abuse" (305.00). The patient is initially absolved, at least in part, from blame and responsibility; the problem becomes one for the mental health professional to treat. However, the patient must follow the doctor's advice, or the consequences (familial, financial, or legal) might be perilous.

The practical impact of *DSM* on personal behavior, and on social, political, and economic policy can hardly be exaggerated, wrote Szasz. "No psychiatric hospitalization or treatment, no claim for reimbursement for psychiatric services or psychiatric disability, no commitment order or insanity plea is valid unless it is supported by an appropriate *DSM* diagnosis."[21] *DSM* also serves as a "marketing tool." Without a diagnostic category, there is no disease and therefore no need for treatment; with one, there may be a designer drug that was created just for the amelioration of that specific ailment.[22]

In sum, *DSM* named things, and named them with authority. This is an achievement that cannot be overestimated. Sociologists understand that without a name, a phenomenon—real or not—has no social or cultural existence. It cannot even be referred to in ordinary conversation, let alone submitted for an insurance claim. So named in *DSM*, collections of symptoms became official referents, each demanding an etiology, a lifecourse, a research and education agenda, and, perhaps most importantly, a program of treatment by a highly trained professional specialist.

Thus, does the name create (whether in truth or out of whole cloth) the phenomenon. Yet there is an obvious problem: "I learned very early," wrote physicist and Nobel Laureate Richard Feynman, "the difference between knowing the name of something and knowing something."[23]

And let us not forget the not-naming or un-naming of things, which is just as significant. Surely the most publicized change between the second and third edition was over the issue of homosexuality. In 1974, the members of the APA voted (58% in the affirmative) that homosexuality no longer be considered a mental illness. In a published resolution, the APA declared that heretofore "homosexuality per se implies no impairment in judgment, stability, reliability, or general social and vocational capabilities." Furthermore, the APA "urges all mental health professionals to take the lead in removing the stigma of mental illness that has long been associated with homosexual orientation."[24]

Informed by this debate, *DSM-III* came to a compromise: only "ego-dystonic" homosexuality, that is homosexuality in persons whose sexual orientation cause themselves emotional distress, was considered a mental illness. This diagnosis proved short-lived; it was removed entirely in *DSM-IV*.

The APA's decision on homosexuality was an attempt to remove a label and therefore to remove a stigma. The impetus for the change, however, was not a new article in *JAMA* or some other medical journal that reported hitherto unknown findings. Science had little to do with the APA's decision. It was rather a cultural judgment, one that we think was both correct and appropriate. Yet there is an important lesson here. What we learn is that all assessments about what is "normal"and what is not are, at great part, cultural. It would be impossible, and not even reasonable, for *DSM* to be free of such social judgments.

We began this section with the question: Is mental illness really an illness? We conclude, having examined the *DSM*, still not knowing the answer.

Job's Depression
Months of delusion I have assigned for me,
Nothing for my own but nights of grief,
Lying in bed, I wonder when will it be day?
Risen I think how slowly evening comes.
Restlessly I fret till twilight falls.
—The Book of Job, 7:1.6

According to NIMH, "depression" is an illness that "involves the body, mood, and thoughts [which] affects the way a person eats and sleeps...feels about oneself...and thinks about things." Depression is not the same as "a passing blue mood." Nor is it (recall the sociological concept of "sick role" which, in part, removes blame) "a sign of personal weakness." Without treatment, the disease and its consequences can be serious, but "appropriate treatment can help most people who suffer from depression." Depression is categorized as major or minor, the former being when symptoms interfere with the ability to work, study, eat, or enjoy once pleasurable activities. The illness is defined by a series of psychological symptoms, not only beginning with "persistent, sad, anxious or 'empty' moods, feelings of hopelessness, pessimism, worthlessness, helplessness, and so forth, but also "headaches, digestive disorders, and chronic pain" that does not respond to treatment.[25]

We return to Job's lament.

"By today's standards," said Fran, "it is obvious that he suffered from clinical depression, presumably..." she thumbed through the volume, "a 'major' and 'recurrent' depressive disorder, most likely 296.3x in *DSM-IV-TR*.

"I agree. His illness probably was characterized by 'melancholic features.'"

"I don't know," retorted Fran. "Given his conversations with God, he probably had 'psychotic features.'"

Throughout most of medical history, he would not have received such a diagnosis. Until the second half of the twentieth century, depression was actually a rare disorder. Individuals suffering from "nerves," which in severe cases were termed "nervous breakdowns," might have been treated with psychotherapy—which is how Job would have been treated through the first two-thirds of the twentieth century. If drugs were used, they would have been opiates, or later, barbiturates. In the 1930s dexamphetamine were given to patients who suffered fatigue. In 1955, Miltdown was approved for use, followed in the early 1960s by Librium.[26] Valium, introduced in 1963, and called "mother's little helper," in the Rolling Stones song, reached it peak in 1978 when Americans consumed 2.3 billion of the little yellow pills. In the latter part of the twentieth century, "talking therapy" changed, too, as traditional psychotherapy, particularly psychoanalysis, was replaced by so-called cognitive therapy, which eschews deep-seated solutions for practical ones.[27]

With the introduction of SSRIs,[28] everything changed. As we wrote in the previous chapter, SSRIs are now the third leading category of pharmaceuticals in retail dollars.[29] The best known brand, Zoloft, was in

2003 fifth in sales at $2.6 billion, followed immediately by Paxil, which grossed $2.3 billion in sales. Yet another SSRI, Celexa, placed seventeenth in sales, grossing $1.5 billion. SSRIs were also third in prescription activity, 140 million in 2002, up 12.6% from 2001.

It is generally believed that SSRIs are effective in the treatment of depression. Prescriptions are easy to get and millions of Americans take them. But, in this book, we repeatedly ask the question: Do they work? That is, are SSRIs effective treatments for depression?

In the early 1990s, SSRIs were tested against so-called tricyclic antidepressants (TCA), the drugs they replaced. Meta-analysis showed that SSRIs were no more effective in outpatient depression than were the older agents. Side effects of SSRIs, lack of which were a purported benefit, were only slightly less than for TCAs.[30] "Later in the 1990s," according to David Healy, "it became clear that a large number of trials with less favorable results for the SSRIs were simply not reported by the sponsors, the pharmaceutical companies."[31]

One important and different kind of meta-analysis used the Freedom of Information Act to obtain FDA reviews of every clinical trial—published or unpublished—of SSRIs between 1987 and 1999. On average, placebos were 80% as effective as the SSRIs. According to Marcia Angell, the former editor-in-chief of the *New England Journal of Medicine*, the difference between treated and untreated groups "is very unlikely to be of clinical significance." Thus, based on all the evidence, not just what the pharmaceutical companies choose to publish, SSRIs "do not look like the miracle drugs we have been led to believe they are."[32]

The general consensus is that SSRIs seem to be effective, though not greatly, in the treatment of major depression. They would seem to be minimally effective in the treatment of minor depression. For example, one meta-analysis concluded that there was "small to moderate benefit" for the treatment of minor depression. For major depression, SSRIs were "clearly beneficial" though as the authors are careful to note, the efficacy is most easily established "in carefully selected patients."[33]

SUICIDE AND MURDER

A hearing about suicide, and a murder trial, frame our discussion.
The suicide hearing:

15 September 2004—In a 15–8 vote, a panel of experts recommended that the FDA warn physicians and patients in the strongest possible terms

*that antidepressants fail in most cases to cure depression in children and
teenagers; even worse, for every 100 patients given the drug, 2–3 will
become suicidal. "We have very good evidence of harm," said one member
of the advisory panel, "and very little evidence of efficacy." Pfizer
responded that the FDA should remember "the devastating impact of
untreated depression."[34]*

Five months later:
The murder trial:

*15 February 2005—In a story that received national media coverage, a
teenager who blamed the antidepressant Zoloft for his violent behavior
was convicted of killing his grandparents when he was 12 years old.
Pfizer, which has fourteen criminal cases pending, welcomed the decision.
"Zoloft didn't cause his problems, nor did the medication drive him to
commit murder. On these two points, both Pfizer and the jury agree.[35]*

Whatever their effectiveness, one thing is sure: SSRIs are used more
than ever to treat depression in children and adolescents. Between 1995
and 2002, "drug mentions per physician visit" grew by only 29% among
the elderly, and faster for each younger age group; for young people—
age 18 and under, use of SSRIs increased by a whopping 124%. Even
after the controversy began over suicide, sales continued to increase. In
2002, the most recent data available at this time of writing, physicians
wrote 11 million prescriptions—8% of the total for all antidepressants—
for children and teenagers.[36]

According to current definitions, how common is adolescent depression? At some point, about 15-20% of all adolescents experience major
depression. At any given time, prevalence is estimated at about 6%, and
28% of all adolescents report periods of depression during the past year
that led to "impairment." Depression is associated with suicide, the leading cause of death for youth aged 15–24, as well as other problems
including school dropout, pregnancy, and substance abuse.

Are SSRIs effective in the treatment of adolescent depression? The
"TADS" (Treatment of Adolescents Study), the best study to address
such questions, was designed to assess the effectiveness of SSRIs alone
and in combination with talking therapies. The design was ambitious:
439 adolescents (age 12–17) with major depressive disorder were randomly assigned to one of four treatment groups: Prozac (chemical
name, Fluoxetine) along with cognitive therapy, Prozac alone, cognitive
therapy alone, or placebo.[37] Treatment lasted twelve weeks and took
place at thirteen academic and community settings between the years

2000 and 2003. Those receiving drugs were monitored six times; cognitive therapy "designed to restructure the negative thought patterns typical of depression," took place in fifteen sessions. Placebo treatment, which was double-blinded with drug only treatment, received the same six clinical visits.

The findings: given a combination of cognitive therapy and Prozac, 71% improved; Prozac alone helped 60%; cognitive therapy alone benefited 43%; finally, the placebo helped 35%. This sounds impressive, and perhaps is. Yet the actual amount or degree of improvement (measured by self reports of feelings and behaviors, was less impressive. On the "Children's Depression Rating," patients with Prozac and cognitive therapy improved by an average of 23 points; those on placebos improved by 19 points. One more point: TADS reported suicidal thoughts in 7% who took Prozac compared with 4% in the placebo group.

The authors concluded (perhaps a bit defensively) that: "despite calls to restrict access to medications, medical management of [major depression] with Prozac, including careful monitoring for adverse events, should be made widely available, not discouraged.[38] This conclusion received a cautious endorsement—"as is usually the case with good research, the study provides not only important answers, but also raises several important questions"—from a *JAMA* editorial in the same issue.[39]

Other commentators were more critical. Several reviewers pointed out that only 71% of the Prozac group and 54% of the placebo group finished the trial. Who dropped out of the study and why? Were the drop outs more depressed or less? The high rates of noncooperation make any claims of statistical significance, which is based on assumptions of randomness, quite problematic. Without proper analysis of this design problem, which was not given, the authors should not have concluded that Prozac was so effective.

There were other problems, particularly related to the small incremental improvement that SSRIs provided. "We disagree with the [TADS] conclusion," wrote two physicians. Analysis shows that "the placebo effects were 86% of the Prozac effects." This 14% substantive improvement came with myriad adverse physiological effects (diarrhea, insomnia and sedation) as well as higher rate of psychiatric adverse events (irritability, mania, and fatigue). The authors recommend drug-free treatment such as cognitive behavioral therapy or even a psychological placebo such as exercise.[40]

Another critic criticized the study's design, noting that the group which received Prozac with cognitive therapy, for which most benefit was claimed, was not double or even single-blinded. Patients in this group knew that they were receiving the real SSRI, as did their physicians, a condition which surely created expectations of maximum benefit—and made comparison with the other groups less meaningful. "The data do not support the TADS authors' optimistic conclusion. The balance between benefit and harm of SSRI for depression in childhood has yet to be shown to be favorable."[41]

We would rephrase: In the treatment of childhood depression, SSRIs do more harm than good. Harm, of course, includes many outcomes—one of which may be the worst of all. Does the use of SSRIs lead to suicide? Unfortunately, the research findings are confusing and contradictory. Still, we can come to three conclusions. In reverse order of causality, they are:

First, there does not seem to be any relationship, or at least "no clear relationship," between SSRIs and suicide. Drug companies have broadcast this conclusion. We are not guilty, they declare. This finding, according a 2005 guest editorial in the *British Medical Journal* "should encourage doctors to prescribe effective doses of these drugs for [moderate to severe depression]."[42] Well, perhaps. Yet for us a finding that SSRIs do not (or may not) cause suicide is hardly a positive. Many drugs do not cause suicide, at least one would so hope, a conclusion which has nothing to do with their efficacy.

That is not the end of the suicide story. Indeed, the cover story of the February 19, 2005 issue of the *British Medical Journal* poses the question: "Do SSRIs Cause Suicide?" As we have seen, the answer would seem to be "no," but.... Here is our second conclusion: SSRIs are associated with increased attempts at suicide, and third, they are associated with increased "suicidal ideation" (thoughts about suicide). Meta-analysis of 701 clinical trials involving more than 87,000 patients confirms the FDA contention: that compared to placebos, SSRIs double both the thoughts and actual attempts (though not the "successful" completion of) suicide.[43] Why do these drugs cause an increase in the idea and attempt, but not the "successful" conclusion, of ones life? It is difficult to imagine a rational explanation, and sadly, none has been offered.

INSANITY

So far we have focused our attention on depression, minor and major. The former, though debilitating, is probably not a life-changing event.

The latter may be, though more typically it is periodic; those so afflicted may be asymptomatic for long periods of time and lead productive and successful lives. Suffice to say, psychiatrists treat more serious afflictions. Some people suffer from psychotic conditions which permanently alter their lives.

We now consider schizophrenia, the most common of these psychoses.

According to the NIMH, schizophrenia is a chronic, severe, and disabling brain disease. It accounts for about 25% of all first admissions to mental hospitals, and 50–60% of persons occupying beds in those hospitals at any given time. Approximately 1% of the U.S. population develops schizophrenia during their lifetime. People with the disease often suffer terrifying symptoms such as hearing internal voices, or believing that other people are reading their minds, controlling their thoughts, or plotting to harm them. These symptoms leave sufferers fearful and withdrawn. Their speech and behavior may be so disorganized that they are incomprehensible or frightening to others.[44]

This definition, which considers schizophrenia as a "brain disease" is strongly influenced by the medical model. Nonetheless, it seems straightforward, as does it array of symptoms—which should lead to reliable diagnosis.

Were the world only that simple.

In 1973, a psychologist from Stanford University published an unique experiment. Under his direction, eight normal people admitted themselves into psychiatric hospitals. Their symptom was that they were hearing voices. It was a phony complaint, but one which was diagnosed each time as schizophrenia. After admission, the "pseudo-patients" acted normally—that is, they were sane in an insane place. Despite their normalcy, the hospital staff interpreted their behavior to fit the original diagnosis. Routine disagreements were seen as deep-seated signs of personal instability. Boredom was interpreted as nervousness. The pseudo-patients remained hospitalized from 7 to 52 days, with an average of 19 days. Upon eventual release, all were deemed to suffer from "schizophrenia in remission." The opening words of the widely cited article that describes this experiment are really its conclusion: "If sanity and insanity exist, how shall we know them?"[45]

This is only one experiment, and one with an unusual design. It does not meet the requirements of good sampling, and therefore it is problematic to draw any general conclusions, or draw them with surety. Nonetheless, at least for us, it is obvious that the diagnosis of schizophrenia is subjective and difficult.

Given the problems of diagnosis, we ask with what effectiveness is schizophrenia treated?

Unfortunately, we can dismiss talking therapy. Or rather we should say that evidence-based medicine has dismissed both psychoanalysis and cognitive therapy. The former was abandoned some time ago; as for the latter, meta-analysis has demonstrated that it does not "confer reliable benefits for patients with schizophrenia and cannot be recommended for clinical practice.[46]

Recall David Rosenhan's experiment. Were it repeated today, his pseudo-patients would surely be treated with drugs (as would Job!), either "neuroleptics," or "atypical antipsychotics."[47] Their common usage is demonstrated by the fact that in 2003, antipsychotics were the sixth leading category of drugs in retail sales.

A word of caution: evaluation of these drugs is difficult. In addition to the problems raised in our discussion of double-blinded studies of depression,[48] it turns out that patient nonadherence rates are very high. In other words, on average about one-third of all patients stop taking their medications,[49] probably because of real or perceived (is there any difference?) side effects such as movement disorders, weight gain, or emotional dullness. These drop-out rates make statistical generalizations, the goal of randomized and blinded studies, almost meaningless.

Neuroleptics (Thorazine, approved for use in 1954, was the first one) are called "first generation" antipsychotic drugs. After six to eight weeks of treatment, about 20% of all patients have a complete remission of their symptoms. Approximately 30% of all treated patients experience a relapse within two years, compared with an 80% relapse rate without treatment. One meta-analysis found that they provide "modest to moderate gains in multiple cognitive domains."[50] The problem is that prolonged use often results in symptoms (involuntary movement, tremors, facial grimaces, etc.) that are similar to Parkinson's Disease. These symptoms may fade slowly, but often they are irreversible. Thus, do these new symptoms, the result of adverse effects of neuroleptics, create a significant medical problem. One other major problem: sudden death, usually from cardiac arrhythmia, is about double that of a healthy population.

Atypical antipsychotics are referred to as second generation drugs. Their widespread use is well documented; in 2003, Zyprexa (chemical name, olanzapine), was sixth in retail sales in the United States. The advantage of second generation drugs is that they have fewer side effects, especially those that produce the dreaded Parkinson-like symptoms. The problem is that 39% of all patients develop agranulocytosis (a decrease in white blood cells)[51] which leads to death in about 1.3% of all cases. Other problems include increases in diabetes and significant weight gain.

All this considered: Are they effective in treatment? Various studies claim that atypical antipsychotics are superior to placebo, but this assessment is statistical rather than clinical significance. Unfortunately, the scientific evaluations of these drugs has produced ambiguity and confusion. According to one study, "there is no evidence to support or refute...." Pardon us, but the translation of this sentence is that there is no evidence that the drug works. We can say no more than the author of one metaanalysis: "The extent to which second-generation antipsychotic agents improve cognition in patients with schizophrenia is controversial."[52]

WHAT IF?

What if the treatment of mental illness disappeared?

Thus far in this chapter, we have seen logic stood upon its head.

Consider clinical depression, the most common of the mental illnesses. Until recently it was an uncommon diagnosis. Since the development of SSRIs, the diagnosis of depression has increased a thousandfold! The NIMH estimates that in any given one year period, 9.5% of the population, or about 19 million American adults, suffer from a depressive illness. Rates are now similarly high for youth.

Why so much depression? Why so much treatment with SSRIs? According to a British psychiatrist: "Reification of biomedical diagnosis acts as a 'justification' for the use of SSRIs in the treatment of childhood depression."[53] If a treatment is available, physicians will find patients who suffer the disease! And find them they do, actually by the millions. "Make no mistake about it," writes one critic, "every prescription written for powerful, mind-altering psychiatric drugs is a government backed experiment."[54] Indeed the relationship between the pharmaceutical industry and the medical community is at the heart (should we say brain?) of the matter. "The way to sell drugs," according to one bioethicist, "is to sell psychiatric illness."[55] According to the clever *New York Times* columnist, Maureen Dowd: "The more anxious the companies feel about profit, the more generalized the generalized anxiety get."[56]

This story contains a profound lesson for our book.

It is easy, and not incorrect, to blame the medical community— from pharmaceuticals to practicing physicians—for this state of affairs. Yet there is more. Another British psychiatrist posited a sociological explanation for adolescent depression. "Whereas prior generations prepared children for the workplace within a society of scarcity," today's children have much higher expectations, "being reared to become pleasure seeking consumers in a prosperous new economy." That along with the increased number of divorces and two working parents leads to much less parental supervision, and such symptoms as irritability, running away from home, decline in schoolwork, and headaches that are all characteristics of what is called "depression." Yet the very label of depression may lead to treatment with SSRIs that does not help and even creates harm. The problem is that we confuse depression with unhappiness, and there is most likely a "genuine increase in the amount of unhappiness" experienced by today's children."[57] The diagnosis of depression is therefore leading the profession of psychiatry into "silences about context, [and] minimizing the real life experiences, stories and strengths of the clients that we see."[58]

In other words, we have medicalized unhappiness. And what is true for adolescents is also true for adults that they come to be. "The fuckin' regularness of life is too fuckin' hard for me," said Tony Soprano in a universal complaint about existential meaninglessness. Tony's basic problem is that "he regards his very being as an inconsequential nothingness."[59]

What is true for depression is true, at least to a degree, for other mental illnesses. "Mental illness is a myth," wrote Thomas Szasz three and a half decades ago, "whose function is to disguise and thus render more palatable the bitter pill of moral conflicts in human relations."[60] Szasz is not saying that suffering does not exist, but rather that the label, "mental illness" actually disguises the problem.[61]

Life is not easy. From time to time, each and every one of us becomes unhappy. Some people, perhaps for reasons outside their control, perhaps not, suffer more than their share of unhappiness. It follows that for most people, this perfectly normal (or at least expected) suffering of the human condition should not be treated with powerful and even dangerous drugs.

For all the time and money and effort put into the treatment of mental illness, little has been accomplished. Few lives are saved. Not many are improved. An entire culture has come to rely on drugs to keep them happy.

Thus, our conclusion: were psychiatry and its related disciplines and professions to disappear, not much would change, at least in terms of mortality and morbidity.

7

MIND-BODY

in which we explore the strange world of placebos and mind-body medicine, and explore the possibility of an expanded medical model

Recall our discussion from chapter 1, in which we decided to disappear mind-body medicine along with the other major specialties. It is surely the case that the bulk of data in this chapter comes from research conducted by physicians; that alone has created an argument for the inclusion of this chapter in the previous section. Yet, as we will see, the ideas herein are on the fringes of contemporary medical practice. For most practicing physicians, the material that follows is viewed with suspicion at best, quackery at worst. For healing happens *despite the physician,* independently of an elaborate and expensive system of treatment. Physicians want no part of the placebo effect, for it messes up their experimental designs, and worse, it undercuts their authority. The very idea of mind-body medicine lies outside the medical model. For it to be taken seriously would require a considerable reconceptualization of what is meant by the notions of health and illness.

BELIEVE IT OR NOT!

As a kid, I was a big fan of *Ripley's Believe It Or Not!* I remember the man who smoked cigarettes through his eyes, and then there was the one who drove six-inch spikes into his head. That was great stuff! I, of course, believed all of it—or at least most of it. Believe it or not, there is an official *Ripley* web site that recounts all this rigmarole. Browsing it, I learned that *Ripley's* did not disappear with my childhood. Indeed, in 2002, they opened a museum in Kuala Lumper. Now all the Malaysian kids can see firsthand what I learned as a child.

> Researching this chapter, Fran and I were reminded of *Ripley*. For example...
> The man who underwent fake surgery but got better...
> The woman who conquered her terminal breast cancer just by talking about it...

Ripley never did statistics, but we can't resist this story, which, if replicated with other cultures and other diseases, would stand contemporary medicine on its head. It goes like this: Chinese Americans with lymphatic cancer who were born in "earth years"—and consequently were deemed by Chinese medical theory to be especially susceptible to diseases involving lumps, nodules, or tumors—had an average age at death of 59.7 years. By contrast, age at death of Chinese Americans born in other years, and nonetheless diagnosed with lymphoma, was 63.6 years. Anglo Americans who have lymphoma were not subject to these calendar effects.[1]

Much of the research in this chapter reminds us of *Believe it or not!*

PLACEBOS

The cure for headache, said Socrates, "was a kind of leaf, which required to be accompanied by a charm, and if a person would repeat the charm at the same time that he used the cure, he would be made whole; without that charm the leaf would be of no avail."

Today we call the leaf a "placebo." By itself it has no effect whatever. For the leaf to have curative powers, the accompanying charm must be administered by a qualified charmer, one who the patient trusts. In today's society, this would be a physician, surrounded by the appurtenances (from stethoscope and white coat to the entire hospital complex) of his or her profession. In its entirety, we call this interaction between patient, leaf, and charm, "the placebo effect."

In our attempt to understand this very real and important and powerful phenomenon, we consider the placebo's effectiveness, definition, and mode of action.

Effectiveness. A British study updates Socrates. In it, 834 women who regularly used analgesics for headache were randomly assigned to one of four groups. The first received aspirin labeled with a widely advertised brand name. The other three groups received the following: the same aspirin in a plain package, a placebo marked with the brand name, and an unmarked placebo. What happened? The branded aspirin worked 64% of the time, followed by the unbranded aspirin, followed by the branded placebo. The unbranded placebo showed the least efficacy, but still worked in 45% of all cases.[2] What are the lessons for this chapter? First, aspirin does work, almost two-thirds of the time—or so it would seem. Second, the placebo worked almost half the time. Third, and most important, the real aspirin worked only 21% more often than the fake stuff.

"I've got a headache from reading all this," I complained.

"I've got just the treatment for it," answered Fran, reaching for the sugar bowl.

"It doesn't work without a white lab coat," I muttered.

And not just headaches. Placebos have proved to be effective treatment in maladies that range from depression and congestive heart failure to gastric ulcer and angina pectoris. They "relieve pain better than anything else,"[3] although this effect is dependent on the context of the treatment. One study of migraine headaches found that placebo injections worked significantly better than placebo pills.[4]

Consider placebo surgery. In chapter 3, we reviewed two dramatic examples—ligation of the mammary artery and arthroscopic surgery. In both cases, fake surgery (cut the skin, but do not alter what's underneath) worked just as well as the real procedure. There are many other examples of successful sham surgery. In exploratory surgery for lumbar disc disease, 37% of the patients reported complete relief from sciatica, and 43% found complete relief from pain—although the surgeon had found no disc herniation—that is, the surgeon did "nothing" (at least with the scalpel) to relieve the patient's pain.[5]

While we might allow the notion that a fake pill can work, sham surgery would seem to be beyond the pale. Yet the phenomenon should not baffle us. Surgeons are among society's elite. They are seen, in popular culture, as icons; their words are taken seriously, their actions (e.g., cutting into the body) are symbolically powerful. Blood itself is transcendental, with complex and myriad meanings—including religious ones—beyond its function as a body fluid. "The shedding of blood is inevitably meaningful in and of itself." In addition, surgical procedures usually have a compelling rational explanation, which drug treatments often do not. The logic of arthroscopic surgery ("we will clean up that messy joint") is much more sensible and understandable, "especially for people in a culture rich in machines and tools," than is the complex but obscure logic of many drugs. Whatever the reason, one thing is sure: sham arthroscopic surgery actually works.[6]

The placebo effect is dependent on the conditions under which the inert substance is administered. It is weakest in double-blinded studies, where the patient has doubt about the medication he or she is taking. Informed consent for any drug, or for sham surgery, reduces its effectiveness. Did I get the treatment? Did I not? The patient must believe—not doubt—the potency and the surety of the treatment. The placebo effect is higher in single-blinded studies, where there may be all sorts of cues about the nature of the medication, and highest in uncontrolled clinical trials where treatment was thought to be effective, but subsequently found ineffective. "Surgery is especially prone to placebo effects, since controlled studies are not required by government agencies"[7] A treatment for angina pectoris that was later found ineffective reported improvement in 82% of all patients.[8] Thus, ironically, we have labeled a treatment as useless, though it helped more than four of five patients!

Definition. These findings, which seem to fly in the face of the medical model, are not easily explained. Nor is the term "placebo," easily defined. One older but succinct definition is that a placebo is "any effect attributable to a pill, potion, or procedure, but not to its pharmacodynamic or specific properties."[9] Or this: the placebo is a

> pharmacophysiological process in which the patient's belief in or
> anticipation of recovery can influence specific biological parameters
> to counteract somatic dysfunction or pathology (specific effects) or,
> by relieving anxiety or pessimism, leads to the alleviation of symp-
> toms (nonspecific effects)[10]

Yet another definition emphasizes the clinical context of the placebo, including such physician behaviors as: "The communication of concern, monitoring and diagnostic procedures, labeling or explanation of the disease, and, more importantly, the impact of factors such as expectation, hope, and anxiety reduction."[11]

Explanation. We say that the placebo is powerful. But that is sloppy thinking. Of one thing we can be absolutely certain: by themselves, placebos are inert. "Placebos do not cause the placebo effect."[12] They cause nothing.

The placebo effect is better thought of "as an effect of the relationship between patient and doctor."[13] We might think of the placebo effect as a drama with three actors: the physician, the placebo, and the patient, in which the patient plays the starring role.[14] As a play is life's imitation, the actors speak not just to the audience, but as well to one another. The doctor-patient discourse is not a neutral factor in the patient's prognosis. For example, the physician's diagnosis not only directs the course of treatment, but it also is itself treatment. For the patient, the diagnosis itself may provide hope that stimulates a healing effect. Or, as in the case of a cancer diagnosis, it might provide a death sentence. Whatever the effect, "belief and meaning are at the center of the therapeutic encounter."[15]

Perhaps the best way to think about placebos is that they are ritualized healing, in which an object with symbol meaning initiates a complex set of effects, be they physiological, neurological, or immunological. Those symbols may be behaviors or spoken words, or even written words. In the classic study of aspirin, it seems that the aspirin label works independently of the drug inside the bottle. In other words, what is working is just words. At first, this position seems ridiculous. Yet we should not dismiss the significance of words, written or oral. One who does not believe in the power of rhetoric is one "who has never been told 'I love you.'"[16]

Not just words, but actions, or at least presumed actions, can be placebos. In common sense, sham surgery cannot in and of itself be a beneficial effect. But it does, and contemporary scientific medicine must deal with that finding.

In the past decade, researchers have gained some understanding of the physiology of the placebo effect. It is known, for example, the placebos stimulate the body's own natural opiates, called endorphins, which will alleviate pain. Other work has shown that placebos can actually activate the body's immune system. An explication of this work goes beyond the scope of this book. Suffice it to say that such knowledge of the placebo effect would shed light on important medical issues.

Yet the issue of causation remains: whether it is endorphins or the immune system or other mechanisms or some combination of these, healing begins with what has been called a "meaning response."[17]

Let us conclude this section with an evaluation of the placebo's place in contemporary medicine. In previous chapters, we've mentioned the word this phenomenon on several occasions, but almost always as an afterthought or footnote to a study that assesses some therapy. Given its evident healing power that we reviewed above, why is the placebo considered at the margins of medicine?[18] To address that question, we need to consider the method of evaluation and proof in clinical studies.

The gold standard of any evaluation is the randomized double-blinded trial.[19] Clinical effectiveness is calculated by subtracting the placebo effect from the experimental effect. The difference, and only the difference, is attributed to that which is being studied. The more the placebo accomplishes, the less can be credited to the experimental treatment. It follows that those who design clinical trials would hope for a very small placebo effect, for it only gets in the way—muddies the waters—of the "real" effect, the one they are looking for, hoping to publish, and hoping to save lives. For clinicians, then, the placebo "is tolerated as a necessary nuisance" but is otherwise "considered with contempt."[20]

Thus, our point: given this marginal status, the placebo effect is an unlikely beacon of light to illuminate the forest of our ignorance. Placebos can teach us "how far we still are from closure on the question of what it will mean to create a science subtle and complex enough all that is entailed in being human."[21]

Our opportunity is great. We dare not ignore the placebo.

PSYCHE

The placebo effect is but one example of how psychological factors influence health and illness.

Here is the first and only joke in this book: "Where do you hurt?" the gastroenterologist asked the neurologist having belly pain. "In my head, of course!" The joke, which is probably not funny, nicely illustrates the so-called anatomo-clinical gaze, in which physicians believe that pain is associated with a specific body site.

What if we were to edit the joke and for the word "head" substitute the word "mind?" This changes everything. Instead of being associated with a body part, pain is now expressed independently of any organ, structure, or tissue—and also independently of clear definition. For who can adequately define "mind," let alone appreciate its very great mystery? Surely the task is beyond this book, and perhaps beyond any tome. Clearly it has been beyond the scope of medicine. The concept is associated more with theology or philosophy than it is with medicine.

To invoke the mind is to leave standard medical practice behind, replacing it with....

Therein lies the problem and the challenge.

Consider this Italian study: researchers found that when a patient witnessed injections of analgesics, the drugs were significantly more effective in reducing pain than when the injections were hidden. Note that the patient is not receiving a placebo. In both cases, the patient receives standard medication, though in only one case are visual cues present. It is the patient's knowledge of the injection which somehow increases the drug's effectiveness. In itself, that is an interesting finding. Yet there is more. The same researchers showed that naloxone, which blocks the body's natural opiates, greatly reduced the open-injection effect. Thus, we have an interaction between an active patient's mind and a physiological pathway. "We are beginning to understand what happens in the patient's brain when he or she interacts with his or her therapist," said one of the study's authors.[22]

As the intrepid commentator, Bill Moyers, wrote:

> If you accept the premise that the mind is not just in the brain but that the mind is a part of a communication network throughout the brain and body, then you can start to see how physiology can affect mental functioning on a moment-to-moment, hour-by-hour, day-by-day basis, much more than we give it credit for.[23]

The notion that the psyche (mind) and soma (body) are not separate entities is not new. Indeed the concept was for most of history (and prehistory) the cornerstone of medical treatment. In the past few decades, there has been renewed interest in so-called mind-body medicine, defined as "interventions that use a variety of techniques designed to facilitate the mind's capacity to affect bodily function and symptoms."[24] Common mind-body treatments include relaxation, meditation, imagery, hypnosis, and biofeedback.[25]

We might assume that psychological problems, such as those reviewed in the previous chapter, are amenable to such therapies. These problems are, after all, all in one's head. Indeed, mind-body treatments have shown some effectiveness in treating psychological problems. So have mind-body therapies been effective in the relief of pain. Once again, we might (incorrectly) dismiss or minimize these claims, given the subjective nature of pain. Yet, according to a major review, there is "considerable evidence of efficacy" in the treatment of disparate maladies such as cardiac rehabilitation, symptoms from cancer and the treatment of cancer, and postsurgical outcomes; and "moderate evidence of efficacy" for the treatment of hypertension and arthritis.[26]

BREAST CANCER

Headaches ache, and pain hurts, and the amelioration of these and other maladies are significant contributions to a healthful life. We do not in any way wish to minimize such accomplishments. Nonetheless, in previous chapters we have insisted on an assessment based on mortality. Moreover, as we argued in chapter 1, we can only assess what has been studied. For these two reasons, we now consider the role of psychosocial factors on the chances of getting, and then the subsequent treatment, of breast cancer.

Incidence

In 2003, researchers from Finland published an article with a significant claim: that stressful life events increase the risk of breast cancer.[27] The design was epidemiological; the method, interestingly, was prospective.[28] In 1981, researchers gave questionnaires to 10,808 women. They were shown a list of stressful life events and asked if they had experienced any of them in the past five years, that is, between 1976 and 1981.[29] The researchers then maintained intermittent contact with these women. By 1996, 180 had developed breast cancer. Women who years earlier had experienced five life events had a 1.31 "hazard rate" (compared to 1.00 for the general population of women with similar characteristics) of getting breast cancer. Women who had been divorced or lost a husband (again, between 1976 and 1981) had hazard ratios of 2.23 and 1.64, respectively.

In addition to the usual controls for economic status and obvious behaviors (smoking, drinking), the Finnish study had an additional design advantage. As part of a larger research project on twins, researchers were able to compare women with breast cancer with their twin pair that did not have the disease. Because the twins share all or half of the genes with their pair, and because most had the same childhood environment, the effect of stressful life events is particularly evident. Thus, the conclusion: stressful life events increase the risk of breast cancer fifteen years later.

These findings were *not* corroborated in the Nurses Health Study, which followed 37,562 U.S. female nurses from 1992 to 2000. More than 1,000 developed invasive breast cancer, but researchers found no relation between job stress and the risk of breast cancer.[30]

How do we reconcile the differences between the Finnish and the Nurses studies? Both had prospective designs, which give each study great strength. The Finnish study had at least two advantages over the Nurses study. First, it assessed all types of life-events stress, whereas the Nurses study was limited to job-related stress. First, the latter considered only job-related stress, whereas the former assessed all types of "life-events" stress, surely a better design. Second, the Finnish study had the advantage of comparing and contrasting twins, and thus, to an extent, minimizing the independent influence of genetic factors. So perhaps we should lean toward the validity of the Finnish study. Yet two previous studies (cited by both the Nurses and the Finnish researchers), both smaller and with less powerful designs, found no relation between stress and breast cancer risk. This would seem to tip the scales toward the Nurses study. Yet as we have maintained throughout this book, any given study, no matter how impressive, should never be used to draw a significant conclusion. A wiser course of action would be to wait for further studies which either confirm or deny whether stress really causes some cancers.

Treatment

We have seen that psychosocial factors might be involved in the incidence of cancer. Is there any evidence that these same factors can influence the course of the disease, or, more specifically, cancer mortality?

In 1976, Stanford Psychiatrist, David Spiegel, designed an experiment to see if he could help women cope with the suffering of terminal breast cancer. Women were randomly assigned to two groups: in addition to standard medical therapy, one group received weekly group therapy, learned relaxation techniques, and were taught self-hypnosis; the other received the same medical care, but no therapy. The experiment succeeded: women in the experimental group reported less pain and stress. In itself, this was a noteworthy finding.

Ten years later, with mind-body notions in vogue, Spiegel examined what happened to the women from the two groups. Much to his surprise, he found that women in the treatment group lived twice as long, an average of 18 months longer, than those in the control group.[31] After four years, one-third of the women in the support group were alive—and two women were still alive fifteen years after intervention; in the control group, all had died. Spiegel concluded that "the therapy seemed to influence [women's] bodies to fight back physically."[32]

These astonishing results, which were widely publicized,[33] held great hope and significance for terminal cancer patients.

Were the world of science that simple. In the years since Spiegel's original study, there have been many attempts to replicate his findings. Most have found that psychosocial support improves mood and self-esteem, and provides some pain relief. Again, this itself is a significant finding. But what about longevity? At least five clinical trials, in varying degrees, have supported Spiegel's original study. At least six others have not. In one of these studies which found no survival benefit,[34] Dr. Spiegel was involved in training and then monitoring all the therapists. The principle investigator of that clinical trial wrote an editorial in the *Journal of Clinical Oncology*, in which she concluded that recent negative findings are "nails in the coffin for potential survival benefits of psychological interventions for cancer."[35]

A month later, Spiegel responded in an editorial in the *New England Journal of Medicine*. One reason for the recent negative findings, he asserted, is that since his original study, "psychosocial support for patients with cancer has improved substantially." Therefore, all patients, even those in control groups, are "less likely now to be emotionally isolated during their illness." It is well-documented that the "secrecy that surrounded cancer in the medical practice of yesteryear undermined rather than enhanced the patient's well being." Thus, one would expect fewer differences between experimental and control groups. Still, the extent to which the mind-body interventions affect disease progression is "ultimately an empirical question." Concluding the 2001 editorial, he wrote: "cancer may not be a question of mind over matter, but mind does matter."[36]

Spiegel's conclusion seems reasonable to us. Do mind-body techniques increase longevity among terminal cancer patients? We don't know. Nor does Spiegel, at least not yet. What we do know are two things about medical science: first, clinical trials are complex imitations of reality; we must expect an array of findings, many of which contradict one another. It follows that scientific progress is rarely a straight road; rather the path to understanding is a crooked one. There is no substitute for replication and refinement—and some patience. Second, this is true for all clinical interventions, including those in more traditional modalities. Indeed, recent medical history is replete with such controversy in the not always successful treatment of cancer.

Spiegel's personal scientific and intellectual journey are instructive. Looking back on the initial experiments on counseling and breast cancer, he wrote: "We never expected to find such an effect. "In fact, I initially followed up on the women in our group because I thought I could *disprove* the notion, popular in the 1980s, that psychological factors could affect the course of cancer."[37] Two decades later, Spiegel had come to doubt his initial hypothesis.

Everyone knows that cancer and depression co-occur. One gets cancer; therefore one becomes depressed. The obverse—that depression could actually influence the odds of getting cancer and the course of the disease—is a controversial idea indeed. Yet in 2003, Spiegel and another colleague wrote that "there is divided but stronger evidence that depression predicts cancer progression and mortality."[38] In other words, there is "a bidirectional relationship between cancer and depression, offering new opportunities for therapeutic interventions."

Even before Spiegel's work, there was evidence that personal factors influenced the odds of getting a disease and surviving it. In a study of 28,000 cancer patients in New Mexico, researchers found that marital status influenced cancer survival. The proportion who survived at least five years was greater among married than unmarried persons, and this was true for both males and females, for all ages, and for all types and stages of cancer. Even among those with advanced disease, married women had a survival advantage over unmarried ones. "The protective impact of being married affected every stage of cancer care," wrote the authors.[39] In another study of women with breast cancer, widowed patients were less likely to survive than married ones, even given similar case histories and income levels.[40]

A NEW BIO-CULTURAL MEDICAL MODEL

In accordance with the medical model, which is the dominant ideology of medicine, the first six chapters of this book have focused almost entirely on the body. This ideology has its roots in the Cartesian division between mind and body. In this thinking, disease is a somatic problem, resulting from injury, breakdown, infection, or inheritance. Curing an illness becomes a matter of the physicians' techniques in changing some aspect of the body's structure (surgery) or function (physiology), or by defeating some enemy of the body, such as bacteria (antibiotic treatment) or virus. In the same way, as we noted in our chapter on mental health, contemporary medicine conceptualizes the mind as the brain, another body part. When the mind (i.e., brain) breaks or deteriorates or is diseased, it must be treated by an appropriate specialist in the same mode (surgery, drugs, etc.) as would any body part that needs mending.

The problem is that the medical model cannot account for many of the "Believe-It-Or-Not" findings in this chapter. How can fake surgery "work," sometimes as well as the real procedure? How can "just" talking help women with terminal breast cancer live longer? Astrology notwithstanding, how could someone's date of birth affect their life chances?

When the placebo effects are large, as we have seen in many different studies, they are "routinely ignored."[41] For who would address the fact that the placebo is 88% as effective (the case with SSRIs) as a powerful drug? The implications, scientific and professional, are profound. Or even worse: when the placebo effect equals the treatment effect, as is the case with sham (placebo) arthroscopic surgery, the entire procedure, 650,000 operations in the U.S. per annum, is called into question.

To believe in the significance of such findings, the clinician would not only need to abandon his or her original hypothesis, but instead to adopt a very different view of health and illness. In the introduction to an interdisciplinary exploration of the placebo effect, a leading authority wrote:

> Placebos are the ghosts that haunt our house of biomedical objectivity, the creatures that rise up from the dark and expose the paradoxes and fissures in our own self-created definitions of the real and active factors in treatment.[42]

These empirical problems lead us to what Thomas Kuhn has called an "anomaly,"[43] that is, a result which cannot be explained by the dominant paradigm, in this case the medical model. Anomalies can lead to one in four outcomes: the model ignores the anomaly and becomes a dogma; the anomaly is discredited, in which case the model endures; the model is expanded to encompass the anomaly, in which case a revised model endures; or the entire model is rejected for a new one that explains the discrepant finding.

The first option is where we are, at this moment, headed. For the most part, clinical medicine ignores or minimizes the findings in this chapter. Such continuance would happen at our great peril. "In science, a model is revised or abandoned when it fails to account adequately for all the new data, wrote a prominent psychiatrist in criticism of the medical model. "A dogma, on the other hand, requires that discrepant data be forced to fit the model or be excluded."[44]

The second option seems unlikely to us. There are simply too much discrepant data. The placebo effect is well-documented. Mind-body techniques are earning their place in contemporary medical practice. The fourth model is probably too radical, in that it calls for throwing away much that is valuable and effective medicine. Who among us is willing to really have medicine disappear?

Our guess is that either the third outcome will prevail. A new biosocial medical model would not reject scientific bioscience, but rather expand its base to include our "Believe-It-Or-Not" findings.

What would be the parameters of such a model? Most authors are vague on this point, and perhaps any indeterminate model should be open to criticism. We don't think so. The medical model was not born overnight, nor would its replacement spring forth quickly. The amount of funding for such research has been so far infinitesimal.

We can outline some of the characteristics of a new biosocial model. First, the boundaries between health and disease "are far from clear, for they are diffused by cultural, social, and psychological considerations."[45] Illness and health are not discrete states, but rather part of a normal and natural continuum. As the brilliant neurologist Oliver Sacks wrote:

> For me, as a physician, nature's richness is to be studied in the phe-
> nomena of health and disease, in the endless forms of individual
> adaptation by which human organisms, people, adapt and reconstruct
> themselves, faced with the challenges and vicissitudes of life.[46]

First, disease, in this view, is a "paradox," with a "creative potential" that must be appreciated to truly understand life.

Second, the doctor-patient relationship must be taken seriously not only as a social interaction, but also as a significant beginning of treatment. Third, the patient, rather than being a receptacle of the malady, is part and parcel of it—meaning that the patient's behaviors, including (as one example) recent incidences of stress, are of great significance in the diagnosis and treatment of his or her disease condition.

It is this different view that needs exploration. Note that we are not advocating a specific alternative to the medical model, but rather we are trying to be open-minded. That there are unexpected and sometimes dramatic findings that need explanation is our beginning. To ignore the placebo effect and mind-body therapies is to snub scientific medicine, and as well miss a potentially great and valuable lesson about health and illness.

8

A WORLD WITHOUT MEDICINE

in which we reprise the findings of this book, consider our
future options, and pose a difficult question

We were on our deck again, finishing a bottle of wine and the
remains of a fine meal in the fading light of a warm summer night. The
trees on the far side of the pond were showing their first signs of bright
color, surely a misleading sign. More than four seasons had passed since
we posed our thought experiment. Geological time notwithstanding, we
were a year older. The issue of our own mortality, never buried too
deeply, had become less easy to ignore—as was the institution of medicine, participation in which is our cultural way of warding off those
demons.

Our thought experiment is a work of imagination, but hopefully it is
truthful imagination.

The huge and influential institution of medicine, one with a central
place in our lives, will not disappear. But what if we envision, as we have
done, a world without medicine? There would be no primary care, nor
would there be surgery, nor other specialties, nor pharmaceuticals. The
medical model as well would disappear. At first glance, the effect would
seem to be devastating. Surely more people would die and die before
their time.

Our thought experiment reveals a different picture.

Most people readily suppose what the AMA purported in 1922: that seemingly normal adults can harbor disease; that examination can detect hidden disease at an "early" stage; and, most importantly, that such discovery can lead to arrest, reversal, or cure, and thereby reduce morbidity and mortality. Thus, do we believe in the so-called medical model.

Most of us assume, and more importantly act on the assumption, that routine physical exams contribute to our health and longevity. Similar is the notion that routine screening for cancer of the breast or prostate, or many other diseases, will add years to our lives. In the same vein, most people suppose that surgery is not only necessary but efficacious, that the performance of both routine and heroic surgeries add years to our lives. Most of us believe that highly touted drugs work, that they protect us from heart ailments or their recurrence or that they stop cancer's deadly metastasis, and in so doing prolong our lives. Most of us believe that mental illness is akin to any other illness and that it can be treated effectively.

Thus, do we suppose.

Yet these suppositions, each of them, are flawed.

Routine screening does find undiagnosed heart disease, vascular disease and cancer. But—as we established in chapter 2—diagnosis does not mean cure. Unfortunately, screening has very little impact on mortality, though its "false-positives" (abnormal results in a healthy patient) surely increase our level of stress—and therefore increase the probability of new illness. Indeed physicians understand the limited utility and value of such procedures, but, amazingly, justify them with the notion that they increase trust between doctor and patient. Such justification, we believe, does nothing less than threaten the legitimacy of contemporary medicine.

Most accept without question the necessity and efficacy of major gynecological surgeries. In fact, some considerable portion of 855 thousand Cesarean-sections and 633 thousand hysterectomies per annum are not medically indicated, and have little if any impact on mortality or even morbidity. Indeed one could argue that such procedures increase human suffering. Similarly we do not question the need for the two most common cardiac surgeries, more than one million insertion of stent or 533 thousand coronary artery bypasses per annum. In chapter 3, we examined the efforts of surgeons, and found that the seemingly obvious benefits of cardiac bypass surgery and stents are maddeningly difficult to demonstrate with clinical evidence, a statement that is strangely and counterintuitively true for many common surgeries.

Surely emergency medicine saves lives. Such a statement, which would seem to have what logicians call "face validity," is difficult to substantiate. Where most lives are saved is not in the emergency room itself, and not even through the direct intervention of highly trained physicians, but through the implementation of what is called the "chain of survival," a system of emergency intervention that begins in the community, is mediated by specially trained personnel (who are not physicians), and terminates, for better or worse, at the hospital.

What about lifesaving pharmaceuticals? Three points are worth noting. First, Americans take an unprecedented amount of prescription drugs, more than ten per person in 2002, a dollar amount approaching one-fifth of total health care spending in the United States. In 2001, prescription medicine expenses accounted for 18.5% of total health care spending in the United States. Second, the most commonly prescribed drug is Vicodin, which makes no contribution to mortality reduction. In 2003, 15.7 million Americans had used the substance, of whom 5 million—according to official estimates—abused it. Third, our most commonly prescribed drugs are ineffective. Despite all their hype, Statins have little effect on the prevention of second heart attacks; ACE inhibitors are no more effective than common diuretics. Finally, many commonly prescribed drugs are not only ineffective, but dangerous. The role of our pharmaceutical industry in overall health care is nothing short of a national scandal.

We are not saying that contemporary medicine does no good. Nor are we advising readers to disengage from the system. As Thomas McKeown, himself a skeptical physician, wrote:

> The conclusion that medical intervention is often less effective that has been thought in no way diminishes the significance of the clinical function. When people are ill they want all that is possible to be done for them and small benefits are welcome when larger ones are not available. Moreover, inability to control the outcome of disease does not reduce the importance of the pastoral or Samaritan role of the doctor. In some ways it increases it.[1]

We endorse McKeown's position without reservation.

That said—and believed—we do not assume the effectiveness of a procedure or drug simply because it is currently standard medical practice. The story of Vioxx and Celebrex painkillers, unfolding as we write, is instructing us otherwise. That tens of millions of women were given estrogen replacements to alleviate symptoms of menopause and make them "feminine forever" is a good example from a few years earlier. A few years before that, 5-fluorouracil, a highly toxic drug, was widely used for the treatment of colon cancer—even though it was known at the time to be ineffective.

What we are saying is that the medicalization of our lives—test this, monitor that, cut this, drug that—has a minimal impact on mortality. As long as medicine focuses on the treatment of illness, rather than on the maintenance of health, the results of its mighty and heroic (and expensive) efforts will be minimal. Short-term efforts at the end of a long process are inevitably less efficient and less effective than one might hope.

The previous six chapters have shown an unexpected picture. We have adopted a way of life that is not too healthful. Rather than vigilance in promoting longevity, our vigilance is directed toward looking for (and also in creating) disease. Seek and (with great effort and expenditure) ye shall find. But what good does finding do? Suffice it to say: though medicine accomplishes much, it is still less than one might think. More specifically, medicine's role in reducing mortality—in saving lives—is less than one might hope.

These lines could conclude our book.

Yet one more task remains.

With medicine gone, what would remain? The task demands no less than a second book. Here we present some preliminary ideas.

ALTERNATIVES

For many years, I took antihistamines for allergies to grass and pollen. I'm not sure if they helped, but they did make me drowsy and dull (and gave me an excuse for the latter). For the past few years, I've taken an extract of nettle leaves. It seems to relieve my allergy symptoms. Fran wonders if the benefit results from a placebo effect. If so, it's fine with me. I'm all for placebo healing.

For the past few years, I (along with about two million other men in the United States) have also taken the botanical, saw palmetto, for treatment of benign prostatic hyperplasia—enlarged but nonmalignant prostate. In 2006, a randomized double-blinded trial of 225 men over age 49 concluded that this botanical was no more effective than a placebo in treating this problem.[2] What am I to do? This is the same as asking: What is the appropriate basis of authority for my (or any individual's) medical decision making?

In 2005, a best-selling book asserted that the medical establishment (pharmaceutical companies and physicians) purposefully keeps natural cures of deadly diseases off the market, that it chooses making money over our health. We don't buy it. Society is just too complex, and power is too widely dispersed in this age of media, to pull of such a massive life or death conspiracy. All it would take is one blogger to break the silence.

What we do understand is that the structure of the economy and its professions is imperialistic, meaning that it seeks to conquer new territory and use its power to hold on to what it has. It follows that the members of the establishment act with great vigor to minimize any nontraditional intrusion into medical practice. It's a conspiracy, but not a legal one! No secret meetings or pacts! Physicians and pharmaceutical executives are not evil people. Their desire to make money is neither unusual nor criminal in a capitalistic society. Still, it is obvious that unorthodox treatments have not received their due—a situation that is unlikely to change in the near future.

Just because the above is true, it does not follow that non-Western and naturopathic treatments cure everything! At the same time, we have little patience for those who claim that all natural treatments are worthless. It is foolish to make any generalizations about a very wide array of non-Western medical practices, from acupuncture to yoga.

VITAMINS

I had just finished my Whopper, large fries, and (of course) diet Coke. My mind's eye envisioned millions of free radicals being released all over my body, each one with the potential of starting a malignancy. Something must be done! This was no time for alternative treatment. Rather with great care and concentration, I took my megavitamin supplement, one recommended by my physician, and washed down with Vitamin C enriched orange juice. Hopefully the antioxidants would prevail this one time, and I would be saved from my own bad behavior. I vowed the very next day to begin eating sensibly.

It is common medical knowledge and common public belief that a balanced diet is essential for maintaining health. Among these essential nutrients are vitamins. During the 1990s, there was a wide acceptance that large supplementary doses of vitamins would not only maintain health, but also mitigate disease.

Vitamin E was supposed to be the poster child. By the mid-1990s, there was considerable epidemiological data which showed an inverse risk between vitamin E intake and cardiovascular risk; the substance seemed similarly active in cancer prevention. The data were doubly attractive, for there was a theory to back it up. Vitamin E, along with vitamins A and C and Selenium, were "antioxidants," that is, they supposedly neutralized the toxic result of oxidation (so-called free radicals) thereby preventing cell damage and subsequent malignant transformation. At the same time they seemed to reduce LDL and diminish arterial clotting, thereby diminishing cardiovascular damage.

It seemed to be too good to be true. By the year 2000, about 12% of all adults (some 24 million people) in the United States consumed megadoses (400 IU) supplements of vitamin E daily.[3] Some 44% of all cardiologists routinely used antioxidants, principally vitamin E, for primary prevention.[4]

Alas, it was too good to be true.

With the turn of the millennium, several clinical trials began to report no relationship between vitamin E, usually at a dose of 400 IU, and either cancer or heart disease. One of those with negative findings was the HOPE (Heart Outcomes Prevention Evaluation) study, a double-blind, placebo-controlled international trial of patients between ages 50 and 75 with vascular disease or diabetes, reported on patients that had been followed for five years.[5] In 2003, after reviewing that study and others, the U.S. Preventive Services Task Force concluded that clinical trials have "failed to demonstrate a consistent or significant effect of any single vitamin or combination of vitamins on incident of or death from cardiovascular disease."[6] At the same time, studies of vitamin A failed to show any efficacy in cancer reduction; indeed, unexpectedly, various studies seemed to show that supplements caused some *increase* in cancer.

There were two possible problems with the HOPE study. First, it was claimed that the time span of the study, 5 years, was too short. By 2005, the HOPE-TOO (On-Going Outcomes), had followed patients for an additional five years, a total of ten years. Their conclusion: Vitamin E did not prevent cancer; nor did it prevent heart disease. Indeed, the study found "an unexpected and disturbing increase in heart failure in patients assigned vitamin E," leading to a recommendation that "Vitamin E supplements "should not be used in patients with vascular disease."[7] The authors conclude with an admonition: that we should not accept the safety of "natural products" (e.g., vitamins), especially if they have not been proven effective.

The HOPE findings, along with other studies, have produced some definitive official judgment. "In 68,000 patients studied to date," wrote the editor of *JAMA* in 2005, "there is no compelling evidence that higher doses of vitamin E reduce cardiovascular risk or cancer; there are even some hints that vitamin E, in excess of normal daily intake, may slightly increase the risk of ischemic events or of heart failure."[8] Added to this is the judgment of the editors of the *Annals of Internal Medicine*: "We think that high-dosage vitamin E may increase overall mortality. Therefore we believe that high-risk and healthy people should avoid this vitamin at high doses."[9]

The second criticism of the HOPE study was that its subjects were sick people, therefore not addressing the claim that vitamin E may prevent illness—the distinction we made previously between primary and secondary prevention. This concern was addressed by the Women's Health Study, which followed almost 40,000 "initially healthy" women at least 45 years of age between the years 1992 and 2004. The findings: 600 IU of vitamin E every second day had no effect on cancer, nor on heart attacks, nor on total mortality. There was, however, a significant 24% reduction in cardiovascular death, and a significant 26% reduction of cardiovascular deaths among those 65 years or older. Particularly evident were fewer sudden deaths among those who received vitamin E.

Despite this unexpected finding, the authors of the Women's Health Study do "not support recommending vitamin E supplementation for [the prevention of heart disease] or cancer among healthy women." Rather they promote "therapeutic lifestyle changes including a healthy diet" as the best form of primary prevention.[10]

How do we explain these disappointing and unexpected results? We might think that supplementary pills cannot substitute for nutrients in natural foods. Common sense would support the notion that taking a pill is not the same as eating. Yet, in general, nutritional supplements are highly "bioavailable," meaning that they can be readily used by the body. Nonetheless, nutrient-food interactions are complex.[11] For example, the simultaneous ingestion of fats increases the availability of lycopene and carotenoids supplements. Some vitamins are actually more effective in supplements than in foodstuffs (e.g., vitamin A is more bioavailable in supplement than in spinach or sweet potato). On the other hand, lycopene is more available from eggs than from supplements, and cooking tomatoes increases its availability. The usability of vitamins in food varies with the method of preparation. "Far too little is known about nutrient availability as a function of plant variety and maturity." The old canard—more research is needed—is surely true here.

What are we to make of all this? It seems apparent that vitamin E is not effective in the secondary prevention of heart disease or cancer, or in the primary prevention of cancer. It is possible that the supplement is helpful in the primary prevention of heart disease, particularly in protecting against sudden heart failure.

A SKEPTICAL ADDENDUM

Alas, were that the only disappointing finding. Other widely touted antioxidants have not been shown to prevent disease. At the turn of the millennium, one of the most touted supplement was omega-3 fatty acids, found in high concentrations in fish oil. It was widely believed to be a powerful antioxidant that protected against cancer. Alas, a review published in 2006 found no evidence that this supplement was related to the incidence of that dread disease.[12]

Even more: taken-for-granted beliefs about dietary practice have not held up to scientific scrutiny. According to the "Women's Health Initiative," a low fat diet, long a mantra for good health, seems not to prevent breast cancer, colorectal cancer, or cardiovascular disease.[13]

In some academic circles it is fashionable to debunk science. Fair enough. Our thought experiment joins in that effort. But in those same circles, it is fashionable to assume, a priori, that some natural curative is efficacious. We would propose a healthy dose of skepticism, and even more, an agnostic skepticism. Nothing works until it is so demonstrated. to paraphrase T. H. Huxley, the great tragedy of science is that one can slay a beautiful hypothesis with an ugly fact.

ACTUAL CAUSE OF DEATH

In this book, our focus has been on mortality. As we argued in chapter 1, mortality is not only the most easily quantified and objective, but also the best, measure of medicine's efficacy. It is usually stated that the two leading causes of death in the United States are cardiovascular disease and cancer. Yet we reviewed a significant article published in *JAMA* in

2004. Therein, the authors posed a different question: What actually causes one to die of heart disease or cancer—or any of the other leading causes of death?

The leading "actual" causes of death are tobacco followed by obesity, accounting, respectively for 18% and 16% of all deaths.[14] The implications of this finding—for medical practice, research, and public policy— are a book in itself. Here we briefly present the argument.

The case against cigarette smoking is well-known. Smoking is the single most preventable cause of premature death in the United States. Each year, about 438,000 Americans die from cigarette smoking, a loss of about five million years of potential life span, associated with an annual cost of $92 billion in productivity loses. One in every five deaths is smoking related.[15] These mind-boggling numbers overwhelm any potential health gain from the various procedures and treatments reviewed in our first seven chapters.

A related and serious public health problem, and a generally over-looked one, is the effect of secondhand smoking.

Each year, exposure to secondhand smoke causes approximately 35,000 deaths from heart disease, 3,000 deaths from lung cancer. Smoking during pregnancy causes an estimated 910 infant deaths.[16] Evidence is rapidly accumulating that the cardiovascular system is "exquisitely sensitive" to the toxins in secondhand smoke. "The effects of even brief (minutes to hours) passive smoking are often nearly as large (averaging 80% to 90%) as chronic active smoking." Regular exposure to secondhand smoke increases the risk of coronary heart disease by 30%.[17] Indeed, in 1994, a new medical diagnostic code was created for "exposure to secondhand smoke."[18]

And what about obesity? Our conclusion is obvious: Americans are too fat—and getting even fatter!

In 1986, about one in 200 were defined as "morbidly obese." By 2002, that number had quadrupled to one in 50. Combining that category with "obese," included three in ten Americans. In all, two of every three Americans were defined as "overweight" in 2002. Of all children age six through nineteen, 31% were overweight.[19]

Suffice it to say: obesity, particularly morbid obesity, is associated with cardiovascular disease, cancer, and type 2 diabetes. A longitudinal study of more than a half million adults aged fifty to seventy, sponsored jointly by the NIH and AARP, found that overweight and obesity were associated with higher death rates for all demographic categories. Increased risk was highest for those who never smoked: death rates were

20-40 percent higher for the overweight, and two to three times higher for the obese.[20] According to one estimate for the year 2000, obesity was responsible for 111,909 excessive deaths.[21]

What has been the medical community's response to this major threat to our health? Alas, it has been tepid at best. As we have seen in chapter 2, the physician is neither trained nor inclined to do personal counseling. Indeed, the medical model focuses on the disease, not the patient, and therefore shows little interest in personal behavior as a causative agent in healthfulness.

One thing the physician can do to combat obesity is bariatric surgery, in which a gastric bypass (about 20% of these procedures restrict the gastric opening) results in significant long-term weight loss. In 1998, surgeons performed 13,365 of these surgeries. By 2002 the number was 72,177; in 2003 it was 102,794, almost an eightfold increase in five years! About 84% of bariatric surgeries were performed on women, a disproportionate amount given that two-thirds of all morbidly obese Americans are female.[22]

What might we expect in the future? It is estimated that by the year 2010 there will be 218,000 bariatric procedures. That number should increase dramatically, given that only about 0.6% of all patients who qualify for the procedure have actually undergone it.[23] These data make us uneasy. Bariatric surgery might be medically indicated in selected patients. Yet we are troubled by a radical surgical solution to what in most cases is a behavioral problem. Better solutions to obesity are surely available.

Nor is gastric bypass without risks. Bariatric surgery is not a regulated or credentialed surgical subspecialty. About 8% of all procedures resulted in complications requiring further surgery. Thirty-day mortality ranges between .5% and 2%. One-year mortality among medicare beneficiaries has been reported as high as 4.6%.[24]

Cigarette smoking and obesity are generally conceptualized as a personal behavioral problems. In a limited sense, this is obviously true. Changing personal behavior can and does benefit one's health. Such change should be encouraged in myriad ways. Yet some critics have gone further, suggesting that personal responsibility for health should be *imposed* by outside authority. Such imposition might be promulgated by employers refusing to hire smokers or drinkers, or by health care providers refusing to insure such people.[25] We understand the impulse. Yet we fear that the proposed cure might be more dangerous than the disease, for to implement such a policy might seriously compromise our rights of privacy, which Fran and I, along with many others, hold quite dear.

Even more, the emphasis on personal responsibility misses the point almost completely. As I wrote some time ago, the decision to begin smoking is one embedded in cultural practices. Yet these behaviors can and have been influenced by government action, particularly the regulation of advertising. Prohibiting television ads, and at the same time allowing antismoking ads, surely reduced the number of new and continuing smokers.[26] The personal really is the political.

The appropriate collective response to the data on cigarette-related mortality is to regulate smoking behavior. In 2004, in private-sector work sites, 8 states banned smoking, but 23 states had no regulations at all; 8 states banned smoking in restaurants, whereas 19 others had no restrictions; 4 states banned smoking in bars, whereas 43 had no regulations at all.[27]

A unique study illustrates the health potential of such legislation. In 2002, the city of Helena, Montana banned smoking in all public places. Within six months, the rate of heart attacks plummeted 58%. For those living outside the city limits there was no change. "We know from long-term studies that the effects of secondhand smoke occur within minutes," wrote the lead physician in the study, "but it was quite stunning to document this large an effect so quickly."[28] Alas, the Montana state legislature, under pressure from the tobacco industry and restaurant and bar owners, overruled the ban. The result: heart attacks quickly returned to their previous rate.

In a related study, scientists from the University of Minnesota asked volunteers (ones who had not smoked cigarettes in at least two years) to spend time in an environment with secondhand smoke, in this case, a casino. After only four hours, the subjects had significant amounts of a biochemical marker in their urine traceable only to a known carcinogen in tobacco. "This is a logical finding," said the lead author, "we were not surprised by these data. But no one has ever shown this."[29]

Neither should obesity be conceptualized as a personal problem, or at least not *merely* as a personal problem.

In America, the highest rates of obesity are found among lower-income groups. The correlation is probably related to what are termed "energy density" and "energy cost." Refined grains, supplemental sugars, and added fats are among the lowest cost sources of dietary energy. They taste good; in addition they are inexpensive and convenient. Unfortunately, these calorie-laden foods are not very nutritious. They have a high energy density and a low energy cost. By contrast, nutrient dense foods such as lean meat, fish, fruit, and fresh vegetables generally have a lower energy density and a higher energy cost. This is all a way of saying the obvious: the less money one has, the less healthy is one's diet. Thus, the growing problem of obesity lies with the "growing disparities in income and wealth, [and the] declining value of the minimum wage" Evidence is emerging "that obesity in America is largely an economic issue.[30]

Recall our discussion from chapter 5 of statins, the drug of choice in preventing heart attacks. According to one meta-analysis that we reviewed, statins reduced heart attacks and strokes by 1.4% compared with the control. In other words, about 71 patients would need to be treated for 3 to 5 years to prevent one such event. There were no differences in mortality between those who took statins and those who took placebos.[31]

We now pose the obvious question: in preventing cardiovascular disease and cancer, which would be the most effective: would it be statins? Or would it be governmental regulation of cigarette smoking or the food industry? To the great detriment of each and all of us, our society focuses on the former. To understand why, we need to pose one final question:

CUI BONO

In the classic murder mystery, the detective solves the crime by asking the question: *cui bono*, who benefits?

In the final section of this book, we ask three questions: who makes money from our illnesses? Who spends money to keep us well? Who makes money from keeping us well?

The answer to the first question—who makes money?—is obvious: physicians as well as any and all connected with health care. In chapters 2 and 3, we presented physicians' substantial salaries. We do no less than put our lives in their well-trained hands and reward them accordingly and handsomely. Again, in a capitalistic society, this is quite understandable. However, our view is different when we turn the tables and ask: How much money do consumers spend on health care. The answer is astonishing. For the year 2004, Americans spent more than $5,000 per capita, which was 14% of the U.S. gross domestic product. More amazing yet: the United States spends far, and a greater proportion of its GDP, more than any other advanced industrial country.[32]

Yet for all the money we spend, what do we get? Very little. We don't live longer than others. Whereas Americans life expectancy was 77.7 years for 2005, the corresponding figures for Japan and Germany were, respectively, 81.2 and 78.7.[33]

A 2006 study comparing the health status of middle-aged people in England and the United States is particularly instructive. This research showed that the U.S. population in late middle age (ages 55–64) "is less healthy than the equivalent British population for diabetes, hypertension, heart disease, myocardial infarction, stroke, lung disease, and cancer." England spends about 40% per capita of the United States total on health care. Yet the authors conclude that "Americans are much sicker than the English."[34]

Thus, do we learn a painful lesson: we are not healthier than others, though we spend an inordinate amount of time and money looking for our diseases in their earliest stages, and though we take more than our share of prescription drugs, few of which do much good.

These findings are a national scandal.

Our second question is: Who spends money to keep us healthy? This answer is not obvious. Let's examine our second most mortal disease. Of the $4.5 billion the NIH spends on cancer research, only about 11% is for so-called prevention.[35] The vast bulk of this money is spent on education for early detection, self-screening for breast cancer being one example. Unfortunately, as we show in chapter 2, this widely practiced screening (as well as most others) offers no advantage whatever in mortality—a surprising result but true nonetheless.

Real prevention, cleaning the air and water, for example, or purifying the food supply, are not even part of the NIH mission. Even worse, our government still pays various and sundry subsidies, actually $345 million in the year 2000, to support tobacco farming.[36] One cannot escape the conclusion that our government fights lung cancer with one fist, just as it promotes that dread disease with the other.

We might focus on the public health establishment. Most of their effort is in controlling some problem that is a manifest threat, say, the spread of infectious disease. This is all for the good, though the effort is tiny by comparison to other branches of institutional medicine. Even so, environmental concerns, even ones that are known causes of cancer, are beyond the mission of the public health establishment.

Finally, our third question: who makes money by keeping us healthy?

Alas, there is no one.

APPENDIX A

ALTERNATIVE MEDICINE

In 1971, Secretary of State Henry Kissinger made a secret trip to China, a country with which the United States had no diplomatic (and hardly another ties) at the time. One of the few reporters in the Kissinger entourage was James Reston of the *New York Times*. During the trip, Reston became ill and required an emergency appendectomy at the Anti-Imperialistic Hospital in Peking. The surgery was successful, but Reston was in considerable postoperative stress. As Reston later wrote, a doctor of acupuncture "inserted three needles into the outer part of my right elbow and below my knees....He also lit two pieces of an herb, which looked like the burning stumps of a broken cheap cigar." Within twenty minutes, Reston noted an improvement; within an hour the pain and discomfort were gone.

This was the first mass media exposure of Americans to acupuncture and traditional Chinese medicine.

"I have seen the past," wrote Reston, "and it works."[1]

DEFINITIONS

The subject of this chapter is known by many names: "unorthodox" or "unconventional," or sometimes less accurately as "naturopathic."[2] In vogue today is "complementary and alternative medicine," abbreviated as CAM. We'll use the term "alternative."

Our first problem is to decide exactly what is alternative? According to one physician, it is "any diagnosis, treatment or prevention that complements mainstream medicine by contributing to a common whole, by satisfying a demand not met by orthodoxy, or by diversifying the conceptual framework of medicine."[3] Perhaps the most straightforward definition is that they are "interventions neither taught widely in medical schools nor generally available in U.S. hospitals."[4] Note that both these definitions define alternatives for what they are not, a problematic reminiscent of the divide between the concepts of sickness and health.

For this and other reasons, the boundary between alternative and orthodox is not well marked.

"The principal distinguishing characteristic [between the two] is their source of introduction," wrote the editor of the *Archives of Internal Medicine* in a special issue devoted to alternative medicine. "American academic medicine has a bias against outsiders."[5] In other words, those therapies that originate inside orthodoxy become conventional; those from outside are deemed alternative. Such is the power of the standard medicine. Or so it seemed. For in the last few decades, the boundary for orthodoxy has become quite porous.

Consider acupuncture and yoga, until a few years ago were considered "unscientific" and alien, their purported effectiveness explained as a result of a placebo effect or hypnosis, or through misreporting or outright lies. Today, along with a host of previously maligned "alternative" practices, they have made inroads into standard medical practice. The editors of *JAMA* now accept acupuncture and yoga as "facts of life," and are encouraging research on those treatments. In 1997, a National Institute of Health Consensus Development Conference concluded that "there is clear evidence that needle acupuncture treatment is effective for postoperative and chemotherapy nausea and vomiting, nausea of pregnancy, and postoperative dental pain."[6] Interestingly, a common site for these practices is on hospital grounds. Our local hospital, for example, has what is called a "*Center for Integrative Medicine*" where one can learn about treatments disdained in the recent past.

TRENDS & POPULARITY

Whatever is meant by alternative medicine, there is no doubt about its widespread use. According to a 1997 survey of the United States, more than four in ten Americans used some form of alternative therapy, an increase from one-third in 1990. Use was more common among women

(49%) and less common among African Americans (33%). Use was higher among those with college incomes and higher incomes, perhaps a surprising finding, considering the labels "unscientific" or "quackery" that are often attached to these practices.

The most commonly treatments were herbal medicines,[7] massage, megavitamins, self-help groups, folk remedies, energy healing, and homeopathy. Alternative medicine was most often used to treat chronic conditions such as back problems, anxiety, and headaches. The authors suggest that some of the above are "more alternative," some "less." In this latter category are biofeedback, hypnosis, guided imagery, relaxation techniques, "lifestyle diet," and vitamin therapy, which, together accounted for less than 10% of total visits to alternative medical practitioners.

Four in ten of these treatments were disclosed to physicians (though we are as always skeptical of such self-reported data), a rate which did not change from 1990. Extrapolation to the U.S. population suggests that there were 629 million visits to alternative medical practitioners, compared with 427 million in 1990. An estimated 15 million adults in 1997 took prescription medicine concurrent with herbal remedies or high dose vitamins.

Estimated expenditures for alternative medicine professional services increased 45% from 1990 to 1997 and were conservatively estimated at $21 billion in 1997, with at least $12.2 billion paid out-of-pocket. *This exceeds the out-of-pocket expenditures for all U.S. hospitalizations.* Total 1997 out-of-pocket expenditures relating to alternative therapies were conservatively estimated at $27 billion, *comparable to the out-of-pocket expenditures for all U.S. physician services.*[8]

APPENDIX B

THOUGHT EXPERIMENTS

"What if...?"

Sociologists routinely pose this question, in teaching, in research, or in the privacy of their own thoughts.

What if at high noon today capital punishment were to be outlawed? Would the murder rate decrease, perhaps because violence would no longer beget violence. Maybe, as conservatives maintain, it would increase with the loss of deterrent punishment? Maybe the rate would remain unchanged, arguably because there is little connection between state and individual action. Each of these possibilities could be considered with theoretical and analytical care, with special consideration given to comparative-historical designs.

What if cigarette sale and consumption were made illegal? Rates of cancer, particularly of the lung, and heart disease would surely decrease; the rate of crime and the size of the criminal population would just as surely increase. Before such a prohibition were considered, it would be worth trying to anticipate with as much rigor as possible what might happen.

Questions are limited only by one's imagination. What if democratic elections were banned in Country "X" or imposed on Country "Y?" Or strict gun control instituted in the United States? What would happen? Or just as important, what would not happen? Each of these in question is surely difficult.

What if all narcotics and opiates were legalized (decriminalized) at this very instant? no legislative process, no getting ready for years, no advance warning for producers and users, let alone law enforcement. What would happen? Just as importantly: what would not happen? Can we learn anything from history, specifically from the experience of alcohol prohibition in the United States? Can we learn anything from comparative studies, specifically the experiences of other countries that have already selectively decriminalized these drugs? That the answers are difficult does not mean that the questions should not be addressed. Indeed, we would assert that had these questions been asked before both twentieth century prohibitions—alcohol and narcotics—considerable misery and trouble might have been avoided.

We might ask even more complex questions: what if an entire institution were to disappear. The very act of asking leads us to think about interesting things. Is it possible, for example, that the state, which after all has (and must by definition have) exclusive rights to the legitimate use of violence, could not even exist without a criminal justice system?

Or what about disappearing the institution of medicine—the subject of this book.

In posing such questions, social scientists are really engaging in "thought experiments," without the label and, as a consequence, without theoretical or methodological rigor. In considering the use of thought experiments in sociology, we are doing nothing more than taking method seriously.

To fully appreciate the possibilities of thought experiments, we need to begin with the classical examples, ones not, as we shall see, constructed by social scientists.

CATS AND CLOCKS

Erwin Schrodinger, one of the founders of quantum physics, had a problem. How could he study the strange notion of indeterminancy that presumably characterized the behavior of subatomic particles? Such behavior not only seemed to violate our standard notions of causality, but was completely out of sight (if not out of mind!). No experimental apparatus could possibly measure and assess such behavior. So in 1935 he proposed a thought experiment—that is, an experiment that is done entirely in one's mind. He invented his famous Schrodinger's Cat[1] and placed him in a black box. Inside the box was a "fiendish" (Schrodinger's term) device which feeds the cat food half the time, and poison the other half. Which one the cat gets depends completely on the random decay of a radioactive sample. In the laboratory is a make-believe "intelligent observer" who ponders the cat's mortality. Occasionally she opens the box. The cat's status, dead or alive, is unknowable unless and until the observer acts. According to the logic and mathematics of quantum physics, Schrodinger argued counterintuitively, it is the observer's act, the observer's measurement, that has determined the cat's status. Thus, Schrodinger used this "experiment" to study the "both/and" characteristics of the quantum world, so very different than our world of "either/or" causality.

This strange indeterminancy was the subject of a rich correspondence between Albert Einstein and Niels Bohr. Imagine a box, wrote Einstein, that can be opened and closed again under the control of a clock inside the box. Apart from the clock and shutter mechanism, the box is filled with radiation. At a predetermined time on the clock, the shutter opens quickly and allows exactly one photon to escape before closing again. Weigh the box before and after, wrote Einstein; the predictable difference will refute the uncertainty principle. For twenty-eight years, from 1927 until his death in 1955, Einstein would compose such thought experiments; in each case, Bohr would refute them with the very practical and mundane details of measurement, in this case, that the box must actually be weighed by a real instrument, which must be suspended on a spring, which must be in a gravitational field, and so forth.

Einstein often used thought experiments. In developing his special theory of relativity, he tried to grasp the bizarre features of objects that travel extraordinarily fast. In one famous experiment, he imagined a train traveling at almost the speed of light, whose engine and caboose are both simultaneously struck by lightening. Place an observer in the middle of the train. Since she is traveling forward, shouldn't the lightening from the engine strike her eyes before that of the caboose? But place a second observer off the train, standing on the tracks. How will she perceive the double lightning strike? In another oft-quoted experiment, Einstein imagined an elevator falling at almost the speed of light, inside which a passenger tosses a ball in the air and watches it fall. Such thought experiments were not only used by the greatest physicists of the twentieth century, but also used fruitfully.

The term, "thought experiment" (*Gedankenexperiment*), was coined by the German physicist, Ernst Mach, who was Einstein's teacher. Thought experiments are not new to the twentieth century. Lucretius used the method to show that space is infinite. "Imagine tossing a spear at its boundary," he wrote. Were the spear to penetrate, it would not be a boundary at all; were the spear to bounce back, there must be something on the other side.

This example nicely illustrates many of the common features of a thought experiment. One visualizes some situation, presumably one that could not be carried out in any laboratory; one carries out an imaginary operation (be it spear or lightning or falling elevator) according to the rules of our everyday world; and one sees what happens. According to the *Stanford Encyclopedia of Philosophy*, "thought experiments are devices of the imagination used to investigate nature."

ISSUES OF LOGIC

All this is interesting, and certainly exotic. Thinking about the method, however, raises an immediate problem: it seems apparent that thought experiments are not really experiments at all. Experiments are designed to answer questions by actions that produce data; thought experiments produce no data. Nor do thought experiments have the characteristics—experimental vs control groups, before and after measurement, *ceteris paribus*, and so forth—that are associated with this design. Real experiments are deeds, not thoughts; they are post priori, whereas thought experiments are limited to the a priori.

Thus, the term "thought experiment" would seem to be an oxymoron. It might be better to think of them as "*controlled* speculation."[2] Nonetheless, "thought experiment" is what this genre is called. It is, after all, a picturesque term that stimulates the imagination; it has a rich history; therefore it is the expression that we use in this paper.

According to one historian of science, thought experiments are arguments, not experiments, that "posit hypothetical or *counterfactual* states of affairs" and "invoke particulars *irrelevant* to the generality of the conclusion."[3] In Einstein's famous examples, there is not and cannot be a train traveling at nearly the speed of light, nor can there be an elevator falling at that rate. These thought experiments began with "counterfactuality." And more: the characteristics of the observer—be she in a train or elevator or, to use another of Einstein's examples, a drugged physicist who finds himself inside a black box—are completely irrelevant to the experiment's conclusions. The observer is not there to observe, but rather to be the focus of a paradox.

Thought experiments typically have three characteristics.[4] They must be *autonomous*, meaning that the experiment's method and conclusion are not dependent on any real laboratory apparatus; they must rely on *mental imagery*; and finally—and interestingly—they must have an element of *bizareness* that appeals to our imagination, that asserts its independence from the real world, and that indicates no intention of execution. Yet, despite these seemingly unrealities, thought experiments are subject to logic. As the correspondence between Bohr and Einstein demonstrated, they can be disproved.

The thought experiment developed in this book meets these three criteria. First, It is autonomous. By that we mean that it need no apparatus outside of our collective imagination; it is not dependent on situations in the real world for its actual conduct. No person must traverse the distance between here and there. Second, it relies on mental imagery—mental subtraction, in this case. What persons or structures will occupy the large empty spaces (physical and intellectual) where medicine once was? It is bizarre. One cannot actually make medicine disappear, let alone any social institution. Indeed—and perhaps this is the point—life as we know it is absolutely dependent upon these complex social inventions.

Whatever we might call them, and whatever their characteristics, thought experiments should be taken seriously as a method of investigation. That is, "they should be studied as if they were experiments."[5] Yet, there are problems with the method. What is one and what is not? Most thought experiments have been used in physics, particularly quantum physics. But other academics have claimed the method for their own disciplines. According to some, much of the Socratic method may be classified as thought experiments.[6] Literary critics claim that utopian novel and science fiction are thought experiments, which seems to us to weaken the rigor of the method. Yet our concern is not what is inside and what is outside an arbitrary border.

Finally, and perhaps most seriously, Professor of Comparative Literature, Richard Rorty, claims that the method is tautological, because it is, after all, our beliefs that determine what we might find imaginable.[7] This criticism is muted, we believe, in the sense that all sociology, indeed all empirical science, must be imagined. How, we might ask, can one imagine anything without some set of beliefs? In that sense, oddly, all intellectual investigation begins with the question, "what if?" and proceeds to experiments of thought.

THOUGHT EXPERIMENTS IN SOCIOLOGY

Thought experiments have found extensive and creative use in physics, particularly quantum mechanics. To our knowledge, no sociological design has ever employed this method. We have been unable to obtain a copy of sociologist Bruno Latour's, "Thought experiments in social science: from social contract to virtual society," the Virtual Society's annual public lecture at Brunel University, 1998. In a personal communication to us, the author asserted: "I have never done anything on thought experiment; if it is not on my web site it does not exist." "Our mistake," we replied in return mail, "was to assume that *Google* is truth. Our faith is shattered."

In considering the use of thought experiments, we raise five related and possibly problematic issues: prediction, complexity, *ceteris paribus*, time-future, and relevance.

Prediction. What sociologists do best is to predict what happens to most people most of the time. Thus, we do not predict the individual event—which one among the married couples will get a divorce on a given day (Will it be the Smiths? or the Jovanowichs?) Rather we predict the aggregate, the probabilities of divorce in large populations. Which is to say: we predict based more or less on the idea of a stable system that exhibits steady change. Such population predictions, we might add, work fairly well.

In this sense, predicting social events is like predicting the weather. From year to year, the temperature is quite predictable. Day-to-day (how many times have we been soaked by the unexpected rainstorm?), it is not. Next year's precipitation is more difficult to predict than next year's temperature, illustrating a general principle of systems: as the number of interactive dependent variables increase, so does the accuracy of any prediction. Still, to forecast tomorrow's weather, an excellent predictor would be today's. On average, the change would be little. In terms of calculus, the instantaneous rate of change is asymptotic to zero. For a slightly better predictor, one would need to know the season, and adjust day-to-day incrementally up or down. Alternatively, last year's weather for the same calendar day would be a good predictor. Other factors are relevant (e.g., long-term trends, including global warming), but one could ignore them with little loss of accuracy.

Our thought experiment violates each and every one of these conditions of prediction. For the stimulus not only happens instantaneously, but it also happens without precedent—and without warning. One moment we have an entire health care system—including our next appointment with the proctologist—the next moment we do not. Perhaps the sociological literature on disasters comes the closest to this idea. The impact of a devastating flood in 1972, for example, almost instantaneously destroyed a way of life in a West Virginia mining town.[8]

Complexity. Secondly, look again at a thought experiment in quantum physics. A cat dines or dies; a lightning bolt hits equidistantly behind and in front of us. The beauty of these examples are that they are not only picturesque, but that they are also quite simple—and quite elegant. Disappearing medicine, by contrast, would be incredibly complex and extraordinarily sloppy. There is so much to consider and far too many variables to control in any reasonable way. Here one has two choices: give up, or, as sociologists are wont to do, glory in the complexity of the world that we inhabit.

Ceteris Paribus. To know what disappears, one must know precise identities? That is, one must have a good map with clearly marked borders. What exactly stays? What goes? *Ceteris Paribus*, always troublesome in any experimental design (more so in a quasi-experimental design where everyday untidy reality intrudes), becomes much more problematic in this complex and messy world. The boundary problem is familiar to sociologists. For example: exactly who is to be considered "middle class?" What are the upper and lower income limits? Is "new" money qualitatively different from "old" money? The very idea of "middle class" raises substantial problems of theory and method, yet as long as we do not fool ourselves, these intellectual and practical issues do not and should not prevent us from routinely using such concepts.

Thus, it is incumbent upon us to define as carefully as possible what disappears and what remains with the disappearance of medicine. This we have attempted in chapter 1 and throughout. When we need to be arbitrary, we should at least understand our own decision-making process.

Time-future. If before the experiment is "t-1," and after it "t-2," then another problem concerns "t-3." That is, what happens at some future time? After medicine's disappearance, one can imagine an expanded role for the clergy. As physicians became the priests of the mid-twentieth century, so might the opposite occur. Various forms of faith healing could become legitimized. Medicine's absence would surely create opportunities for law enforcement. Various other professions would probably expand their borders, particularly—one would speculate—in the areas of substance abuse and mental health.

We do not deny any of these possibilities, but neither do we consider them. We are interested, as it were, only in instantaneous change: here today, gone tomorrow.

Relevance. Finally, the reader might question the relevance of our thought experiment. What is proved? We set the experiment in motion, We go through the mental work of doing it. And then: so what? No one really thinks that drugs will really be decriminalized in the current political climate? Is our effort an elaborate sophistry? One might call my thought experiment an exercise in the social construction of unreality!

Indeed. We are not calling for a less scientific sociology, nor one that is less humanistic. Our aim is a sociology that is not afraid of the imagination—indeed one that incorporates the imaginative into its theory and method with all possible rigor.

UNREALITY

Thomas Kuhn, the philosopher of science whose work has had a great impact on sociology, claimed that thought experiments deal with situations that have not been examined in the laboratory, perhaps because they cannot be examined, perhaps because they do not or need not occur in nature at all. That is, they need not meet ordinary conditions of verisimilitude. Even so, nothing about the experiment can be entirely unfamiliar or strange. Thus, for Kuhn, a thought experiment at minimum can help us understand the scientist's *conceptual apparatus*. Yet they can do more. The paradox of thought experiments is that they often have novel empirical import—even though they are conducted entirely inside one's head. Kuhn asserts that a successful thought experiment can do what an empirical investigation can do—that is, it can help us understand the real world.[9]

Our thought experiment meets the criteria specified by philosophers of science. It is autonomous; once begun, it has a life (or death, as it were) of its own. It is counterfactual; its actual happening is impossible. And it is bizarre; the very thought of a world without Western medicine is difficult to imagine—much more so than one might expect. At this point, it is best to consider our thought experiment as a form of controlled speculation which might expose and inform our own conceptual apparatus. The thought experiment is not real, but no more or less than any work of imagination, or for that matter, any work that is inherently conceptual. We would hope not only for theoretical insight, but also that this thought experiment might, for example, inform the debate on public policy.

There is, it is our contention, only one way to find out. Let us conduct this thought experiment—with all theoretical and methodological rigor—and see what happens?

APPENDIX C

MEDICINE AND MORTALITY

An Historical Perspective

Good mortality data were not available until the mid-nineteenth century in Europe. Yet most scholars conclude that mortality began to decline sometime around 1700. About one-third of the total decline in mortality between then and now occurred prior to the middle of the nineteenth century, and another one-fifth before the beginning of the twentieth century.[1] The period since then—that is, the period of modern medicine—accounts for less than half of the total decline in mortality since 1700.

Before the 1940s, therapeutic successes were few and far between. Whether the patient lived or died was not generally related to the physician's intervention and treatment. "No one, physician or nonphysician would have accorded the lion's share of credit for declining mortality to the personal physician system." With the introduction of sulfonamide and antibiotics after World War II, intervention began to show results. A few patients with acute infections could be cured. There was actually something for physicians to do. "Therapeutic nihilism was no longer the problem. If anything, therapeutic adventurism—the emphasis on cure—rather than care—replaced it."[2]

In the modern era, the decline of mortality has been precipitous and consequential. In the United States, from 1900 to 1973, an historical blink of the eye, mortality declined by 69%. But almost all of that reduction—92%—came before 1950. The average rate of decline from 1900 to 1950 was .22 per thousand, after which it became almost negligible, .at 04 per thousand. Both sexes experienced this decline, which for females leveled off around 1950, while the rate for males actually showed a slight increase from 1960 to 1970.[3]

The real decline in mortality has come at the beginning of life, especially in the first year. In 2002, infant (that is, first year) mortality was 7 per 1,000.[4] It wasn't always so low. Consider this dramatic illustration. For most of human existence, of every ten newborn children, two to three died before their first birthday, five to six by age six, and about seven before maturity. Thus, only three of every ten live births were destined for maturity. Were the infant mortality from the mid-1800s in the United States (which ranged between 15 and 30%) in effect today, each year between a half million and a million babies would perish before their first birthday.[5]

At life's end, there has not been a corresponding improvement. Actuarial life tables for the year 1900 show that a seventy-year-old American, having survived the most dangerous years of youth, could expect to live another 9.3 years. By 1970, a seventy-year-old could expect an additional twelve years, an increased life expectancy of only 2.7 years—the gains being higher for females, lower for males. This is not an insignificant improvement, but it hardly represents a sea change in mortality, especially given the heroic medical efforts often associated with mortality at this age.[6]

Thus, we arrive at two counterintuitive findings, both important for our book: (1) in the past half century, there has not been much decline in the rate of adult mortality in modern societies; and (2) the decline in mortality is not associated with significant increases in life span, or even with large improvements in adult mortality.

Looking backwards from today's modernist, progressive standpoint, the common notion is that the historical decline in mortality is due to the actions—indeed the direct interventions—of doctors. "The genuinely decisive technology of modern medicine," wrote Lewis Thomas, no apologist for modern medicine, "is best exemplified by 'immunization against diphtheria and pertussis [whooping cough]'." The treatment of tuberculosis, he continued, "represents a milestone in human endeavor."[7]

It would seem that Thomas is on firm ground. The research that led to the development of diphtheria antitoxin was awarded the very first Nobel Prize in medicine in 1901. "By the 1930s," according to one historian of medicine, diphtheria had become "the paradigmatic disease of the so-called bacteriological revolution and the symbol of the triumph of scientific medicine in the control of infectious disease."[8] In many ways, "diphtheria was the darling of the bacterial revolution. A disease that had strangled thousands of helpless children every year suddenly became controllable."[9] Thus, were the new powers of medicine.

To believe in science and medicine is to believe in progress, and visa versa. To be modern is to believe that medicine is and must be a science. We will call this way of thinking the *"orthodox position."*

"THE HERESY"

The orthodox answer might be intuitively appealing, but to what extent is it valid? In other words, to what extent are reductions in mortality attributable to the intervention of modern medicine? To answer this question, we turn to the work of Thomas McKeown (1911–1988), professor of Social Medicine at the University of Birmingham Medical School, and John and Sonja McKinley, sociologists at Boston University.[10]

One thing we know: the principal cause in the decrease of mortality has been the reduction in infectious diseases. Since the mid-nineteenth century, according to McKeown, three quarters of the abatement in mortality in Great Britain came from such control. The McKinleys' conclusion for twentieth-century America is comparable. In 1900, about 40% of all deaths were caused by eleven infectious diseases, 16% from three chronic conditions (heart disease, cancer, and stroke), the remainder from other causes. By 1973, only 6% of all deaths were from infectious diseases, whereas deaths from chronic conditions had increased to 58%.

This would seem to precisely the claim of the "orthodox position."

Let us examine reductions in death from diphtheria and whooping cough (childhood pertussis), both airborne infectious diseases, both cited by Thomas "as success" stories of medicine. Both diseases have declined dramatically. Yet 120 years of British data show declines in mortality from these two diseases account for only a small contribution to the total decline in mortality, 6.2%[11] and 2.6%, respectively, together accounting for 8.8% of the total reduction in mortality. Twentieth-century data for the United States tell a similar story. For diphtheria, the fall in the standard death rate as a percentage of the total fall in death rate is 3.6%; for whooping cough it was merely 1%.[12] While these are not insignificant reductions in mortality—each life saved might be seen as extraordinary—neither can they be considered in and of themselves a "great achievement."[13]

The organism that causes diphtheria was identified in the 1880s, and antitoxin was first used—though not widely—in the early 1890s. Fatalities in England and Wales began a precipitous and continuous decline in the 1890s, coincident with the introduction of antitoxin, which would seem to support the orthodox position. Yet there are two cautionary notes. First, fatalities from whooping cough and measles, both with similar natural histories to diphtheria, began a similar decline without a correspondent prophylaxis or treatment; second, the national immunization campaign for diphtheria, which marked the first systematic and widespread use of diphtheria antitoxin in Great Britain, was not initiated until the early 1940s. Still, McKeown notes, that after this national campaign, deaths from diphtheria almost disappeared. Evidence from 1961–1963 indicated that the risk of an attack was about six times greater, and the risk of a fatal attack ten times greater, for the nonimmunized population.

In the United States, use of diphtheria antitoxin became routine after 1930. Consequently, the fall in the standard death rate that can be attributed to intervention is somewhat higher than for other diseases, a success story of sorts. Yet, according to the McKinleys, the decline in death rates after toxoid is only 13.5% of the total decline in mortality from diphtheria, a contribution to the total decline in mortality of only 0.5%.

In England and Wales, the death rate for whooping cough began to decline about 1870, about 35 years before its causal organism was identified. By the time immunization became generally available, mortality was quite rare. In the United States, widespread treatment for whooping cough began early, in 1930, and is responsible, according to the McKinleys, for a 51% fall in mortality. While this is surely an impressive accomplishment, it should be noted that by the 1930s the death rate from whooping cough was already quite low. Indeed these declines in whooping cough mortality account for only 0.5% of the entire decrease in mortality from 1900 to 1970.

Did Lewis Thomas choose the wrong example? Of airborne diseases, the great success story and exemplar of orthodoxy would seem to be tuberculosis. In England and Wales, the death rate from that dreaded disease declined from 2,901 per million in the mid-nineteenth century to only 13 per million in 1971, accounting for 17.5% of the total reduction in standardized death rates. The story is similar for the United States, where from 1900 to 1970, fewer fatalities from tuberculosis accounted for 16.5% of the decline in standard death rate. Yet the story is not so easily interpreted. "It is probable," explained McKeown, that mortality from this disease was falling in the first half of the nineteenth century. In the second half of that century, nearly half the decrease in death rates came from declining tuberculosis mortality.

All this happened long before the advent of modern medical understanding or treatment. The bacillus responsible for tuberculosis was not identified until 1881. Drug therapy was not introduced until the midst of World War II and not commonly used until 1948; BCG vaccine, produced from weakened bovine tuberculosis bacilli, followed a few years later. It is true that in England and Wales death from tuberculosis decreased 51% from 1948 to 1971. Yet this reduction is less significant than it might appear. Closer analysis shows that the introduction of streptomycin barely changed the slope of decline, and that, moreover, chemotherapy accounted for only 3.2% of the entire reduction of deaths since 1848 from that once dreaded disease.[14]

The story repeats itself in the United States. Between 1900 and 1971, reductions in mortality from tuberculosis accounted for 16.5% of the total decrease in mortality. Yet most of this benefit occurred prior to the availability of antibiotics. According to calculations by the McKinleys, only 8.4% of the total decline in tuberculosis mortality can be attributed to modern treatment, and such treatment was responsible for only 1.4% of the total decline in the standardized death rate.[15]

The McKinleys studied the impact of prophylaxis on eleven infectious diseases which had been deadly at the beginning of the twentieth century in the United States. For each one, the authors charted the slope of decline in mortality, marking in each case the first year of widespread medical intervention. The findings are dramatic: for each case the intervention comes long after the most significant declines in mortality. The McKinleys then calculate the fall in the standard death rate after intervention as a percent of the total fall for that disease. The findings are significant. For typhoid, intervention accounted for far less than one-third of 1% of the reduction in mortality; for measles, 1.4%, for scarlet fever, 1.8%. Their conclusion:

> Given that it is precisely for these diseases that medicine claims the
> most success in lowering mortality, 3.5 percent probably represents a

reasonable upper limit estimate of the total contribution of medical measures to the decline in mortality in the United States since 1900.[16]

Thus, do we arrive at a proposition, one that John and Sonja McKinley call the *"heresy:"* that modern medical care is generally unrelated to improvements in the health of populations, or more specifically: that the introduction of specific medical measures and/or the expansion of medical services are generally not responsible for most of the modern decline in mortality.[17]

This is our third, and perhaps most important counterintuitive finding.

McKeown was the first to arrive at this conclusion with data for England and Wales. Except for the immunization against smallpox (accounting for less than 2% of the historical decline death rates), it is "unlikely that personal medical care had a significant effect on mortality from infectious diseases before the twentieth century." Between 1900 and 1935, there were some successful medical interventions: diphtheria antitoxin, surgery for appendicitis, Salversan for syphilis, intravenous therapy for diarrheal diseases, and immunization against tetanus. Yet the contributions of these treatments to the total decline of the death rate was small. Since 1935, sulphanamides and later antibiotics saved lives, but again, their combined contribution to reductions in an already low death rate were minimal.[18]

PUBLIC HEALTH

Remember the case of Sherlock Holmes and the dog that didn't bark? In that story, Holmes solved a mystery because something—a dog which barked at a certain time each evening—did not happen as expected. Thus, what did not happen—what cannot be attributed to medicine—is a significant finding.

If not doctors and their medicine, who (or what) was responsible for the reductions in mortality? This question was considered in chapter 8. For now, we suggest that the principal contribution to the decline in mortality was the improvement in public health, particularly improvements in the quality of food and sanitation.

In the nineteenth century, there were no dramatic changes in working-class living conditions, but there were advances in water purification and sewage control. Beginning in 1900, there were great improvements in food hygiene, especially in the quality of milk. Pasteurization (after

1890), as well as the bottling and safe transport of milk, reduced significantly the incidence of gastroenteritis in infants and children. These hygienic measures were responsible "for at least a fifth of the reduction of the death rate between the mid-nineteenth century and today,"[19] far exceeding the contributions of various "great achievements" in medicine.

"By the time laboratory medicine came effectively into the picture," wrote Rockefeller Institute physician, and widely read author, Rene Dubois, "the job had been carried far toward completion by the humanitarians and social reformers of the nineteenth century." "When the tide is receding from the beach," he concluded with an artful metaphor, "it is easy to have the illusion that one can empty the ocean by removing water with a pail."[20]

And not only public health. As we have seen in chapter 8, lifestyles cannot be overestimated as a causative factor in the maintenance of health—and in the probability of illness and early death. Because people have smoked cigarettes, historical reductions in mortality were considerably less, perhaps by half, than they would have been in a cigarette-free world. Such possible improvements in health dwarf anything and everything done by physicians.

Notes

Chapter 1. Disappearance

1. Editors, "Looking back on the millennium in medicine," *New England Journal of Medicine* 342 (2004): 42–49.

2. Roy Porter, Greatest Benefit: (New York: Norton, 1997).

3. Jason Lazarou, Bruce H. Pomeranz and Paul Corey, "Incidence of adverse drug reactions in hospitalized patients," *JAMA* 279 (1998): 1200–1205.

4. Center for Disease Control, National Nosocomial Infections Surveillance, 1995.

5. L. T. Kohn, *et. al., 1999* "To Error is Human" (Washington, DC: National Academy Press, 1999).

6. Robert Blendonm, et. al., "Views of practicing physicians and the public on medical errors," *New England Journal of Medicine* 347 (2002): 1933–1940. A study of 393 full-time hospital nurses also shows a high error rate. Over a one month period, 30% reported making at least one error, and 33% reported at least one near error. M. C. Balas, L. Scott and A Rogers, "The prevalence and nature of errors and near errors reported by hospital staff nurses," *Applied Nursing Research* 17 (2004): 224–30.

Here is a strange cause and effect. The prevalence of medical errors is related to the decline in autopsies! In 1961, two of five deaths were followed by autopsies, a number that decreased to one in ten in 1994, when the National Center for Health Statistics stopped keeping track of these procedures. Today the estimate is that only one in twenty deaths results in an autopsy. How is this trend relevant to the known incident of medical error? The answer tells us something about contemporary medicine. A study of 1,000 autopsies between 1983 and 1988 found that there were "major discrepancies between autopsies and the clinical diagnosis in 317 cases." While there are many good scientific reasons for doing autopsies, the main reason for *not doing them is the threat of malpractice.* "An autopsy that uncovers an error in treatment also uncovers the potential for litigation," concludes an editorial in the *New York Times*, ("What the body knows," March 4, 2004). Thus, despite the well-known benefits of autopsies, they are avoided lest medical error is revealed.

7. U.S. Congress, House Committee on Interstate and Foreign Commerce. Subcommittee on Oversight and Investigation. "Cost and quality of health care: unnecessary surgery" (Washington, DC: U.S. Government Printing Office, 1976).

8. Quoted in Evelynn Hammonds, *Childhood's Deadly Scourge: The Campaign to Control Diphtheria in New York City, 1880–1930* (Baltimore, MD: Johns Hopkins Press, 1999), p. 221.

9. A. Harris, *et. al.,* "Murder and medicine: The lethality of criminal assault 1960–1999," *Homicide Studies* 6 (2002): 128–66.

10. Two historic and noteworthy changes in cause of death have occurred within the past twenty years. First, there has been a 45% increase in deaths in which diabetes was recorded as the underlying cause (A. Jemal, et. al., 2005). Second, as of 2002, cancer has overtaken heart disease as the leading cause of death in the United States for people under age 85. The reason seems to be a dramatic reduction in mortality from diseases of the heart (American Cancer Society, *Annual Statistical Report*, 2005).

11. All mortality data comes from information on death certificates. Unfortunately, this information is not too reliable. One study that compared contemporary antemortem and postmortem diagnoses showed that the "cause of death" listed on death certificate was incorrect in about one-quarter of all cases. (Thomas McKeown, "Fertility, mortality and causes of death," *Population Studies* 32, (1978): 535.

12. Ali Mokdad, et. al, "Actual cause of death in the United States, 2000," *JAMA* 291 (2004): 1238–45.

13. J. McGinnis and William Foege, "Editorial: The immediate vs the important," *JAMA* 291: 1363–64.

14. Our thanks to Allan Mazur for this suggestion.

15. All quotes from James Petersen and Gerald Markle, "Expansion of conflict in cancer controversies," *Research in Social Movements, Conflict and Change* 4 (1981): 151–169.

16. Gerald Markle and James Petersen, *Politics, Science and Cancer: The Laetrile Phenomenon* (Boulder, CO: Westview Press, 1980).

17. David Eisenberg, et. al., Trends in alternative medicine use in the United States, 1990–1997, *Journal of the American Medical Association* 280 (1998): 1569–1575.

18. Ted Kaptchuk, "The placebo effect in alternative medicine: can the performance of a healing effect have clinical significance?" *Annals of Internal Medicine* 136 (2002): 817–25.

19. The World Health Organization, *The First Ten Years*. (Geneva World Health Organization, 1958).

20. George Engel, "The need for a new medical model: A challenge for biomedicine," *Science* 196 (1975): 129–136.

21. Lone Simonsen, et. al., "Impact of influenza vaccination on seasonal mortality in the U.S. elderly population," 165 (2005): 265–72. The U.S. Centers for Disease Control (CDC), which runs the vaccination program, plans no change in its advice to elderly people. "These results don't contribute to changing vaccine policy," said a CDC epidemiologist." *New York Times*, "Flu shots for elderly may not save lives," February 15, 2005.

22. McKinley, "Refocusing upstream: The political economy of illness," in *Applying Behavioral Science to Cardiovascular Risk* (NY: American Heart Association), pp. 424–425.. The diseases are tuberculosis, scarlet fever, influenza, pneumonia, diphtheria, whooping cough, measles, smallpox, typhoid, and poliomyelitis.

23. Robert Anderson, "United States Life Tables," 1998, *National Vital Statistics Report* 48 (#18), February 7, 2001, Table 11. Life expectancy continues to increase.

In 1998, a seventy-year old American could expect to live an additional 14.3 years, an increase of an additional 2.3 year compared with 1970.

24. Five years before the publication of Illich's book, John Powles' (1970) article, "On the limitations of modern medicine," anticipated many of his arguments as well as those in this book. See also Sol Levine, et. al., provocative chapter, "Does medical care do any good?" published in 1983. Unfortunately neither of these articles are commonly cited anymore. We thank Jim Petersen for making us aware of these two references

25. Illich, Medical Nemesis (New York: Pantheon Books, 1976), p. 1. Ivan Illich was a man who favored the thirteenth century over the twentieth, and who thought that all modern institutions inhibited human freedom. His work was derided by the right, for its suspicion of progress, and the left, for its hostility to the welfare state. He was born in Vienna in 1926. His mother was a Sephardic Jew and his father descended from Dalmatian royalty. Illich trained as a biologist in Florence, then studied theology at the Vatican's Gregorian University, before becoming a parish priest in Puerto Rico. For most of his adult life, he lived in Cuernavaca, Mexico where he wrote numerous influential books, including *Deschooling Society*. He died in 2002 from cancer, which, characteristically, he treated himself.

26. John McKinley and Sonya McKinley, "The questionable contributions of medical measures to the decline of mortality in the United States in the twentieth-century, *Milbank Memorial Fund* Quartely (summer 1977): 401. Thomas McKeown, *The Role of Medicine: Dream, Mirage or Nemesis?* (Princeton, NJ: Princeton University Press, 1979), p, vii.

27. Alvin Gouldner, "The sociologist as partisan: Sociology and the welfare state," *The American Sociologist* 3 (1968): 103–116.

28. Quoted in Ronald Numbers, "The history of American medicine: A field in ferment," *Reviews in American History* 10: p. 251.

29. For a general idea of this new approach to science, see my book with Sheila Jasanoff (who is the first author), Trevor Pinch, and James Petersen, *A Handbook of Science and Technology Studies*, 2d ed. (Beverly Hills: Sage Publications, 2001).

30. John Ioannidis, "Contradicted and initially stronger effects in highly cited research," *JAMA* 294 (2005): 218–28. Ioannidis was quoted in *Newsweek*, July 25, 2005, p. 25.

31. Office of Technology Assessment, *The Impact of Randomized Clinical Trials on Health Policy and Medical Practice* (Washington, DC: U.S. Government Printing Office, 1983).

32. Lewis Thomas, *Lives of a Cell* (New York: Viking, 1974), p. 34.

33. Indeed, the financial arrangements of research have an impact on findings. In a review of 324 cardiovascular clinical trials published in *JAMA* between 2000 and 2005, there were positive findings in two-thirds of the studies funded by for-profit organizations, compared to less than half successes for those funded by nonprofit organizations (Paul Ridker and Jose Torres, "Reported outcomes," 2006).

Chapter 2. Primary Care

1. Only 55% of all primary care physicians were board certified, compared to 60% for all active physicians. One-third of primary care physicians graduated from a foreign medical school, compared with 37% for all physicians. Data on primary care physicians are from Thomas Pasko, and B. Seidman eds., *Physician Characteristics and Distribution in the United States: 2000–2001 Edition* (Chicago: American Medical Association, 2002).

2. Curiously, these data, collected by the American Medical Association for the Bureau of Labor Statistics, are *net income, after expenses*. This figure is different than those reported for other professions (e.g., the 1998 median income—gross, not net—for lawyers was $91,320). What would be the comparable figure for physicians? There is no way to know, but our guess would be two or three times greater.

3. Thomas Bodenheimer, "Primary Care—Will It Survive?" *New England Journal of Medicine* 355 (2006): 861–61. Income data must be interpreted cautiously, depending on the inclusion or exclusion of practitioners of internal medicine as primary care physicians.

4. Data on patient utilization are from Center for Disease Control, *National Ambulatory Medical Care Survey: 1999 Summary*. Vital and Health Statistics 322, July 17, 2001, and *2000 Summary*, Advance Data #328.32, 2002.

5. This is not time spent with the physician. Rather it is the total time in the examination room, either being screened (e.g., blood pressure) by the doctor's assistant, or waiting (nervously perusing a year old magazine) for the physician to arrive, or actually in the doctor's presence.

6. Langewitz, Wolf, et. al., "Spontaneous talking time at start of consultation in outpatient clinic: Cohort study." *British Medical Journal* 325 (2002): 682–683.

7. Joshua Metlay, et. al., "National trends in the use of antibiotics by primary care physicians for adult patients with cough," *Archives of Internal Medicine* 158 (1998): 1813–1818.

8. Caroline Wellbery, "Editorial: Are we prescribing too many antibiotics?" *American Family Physician* 55, no. 5 (1997). The grammatical form of the title, posed as a question, rather than an empirical conclusion, is, for us, questionable.

9. J. Scott, et. al., "Antibiotic use in acute respiratory infections and the ways patients pressure physicians for a prescription," *Journal of Family Practice* 50 (2001): 853.

10. Mitchell Charap, "The periodic health examination: genesis of a myth." *Annals of Internal Medicine* 95 (1981): 733–735.

11. Here is direct evidence of the arrival of the medical model in all its glory. For we were told to celebrate our birthday not by doing something joyful, something life affirming—which might in itself extend our life, but rather by having our bodies probed, prodded and stuck, and in so doing, be reminded (as though a birthday were not enough) that we are all too mortal.

12. Paul Han, "Historical changes in the objectives of the periodic health examination," *Annals of Internal Medicine* 126 (1997): 913.

13. George Rosen, *Preventive Medicine in the United States, 1900–1975: Trends and Interpretations* (New York: History of Science, 1975). One historian argues that annual physicals served the purpose of "enhancing the position of the practitioners in the community, particularly in the wake of their opposition to compulsory health insurance."

14. U.S. Preventive Task Force, *Guide to Clinical Preventive Services: An Assessment of the Effectiveness of 169 Interventions* (Baltimore, MD: Williams & Wilkins, 1989), p. xix. The Task Force was co-chaired by Director of the Division of Primary Care, Lawrence Robert, Harvard Medical School, and Deputy Assistant Secretary for Health, and Director of the U.S. Office of Disease Prevention and Health Promotion, Michael McGinnis, whose office provided staff for this assessment.

15. The most notable example is phenylketonuria (PKU), one genetic condition that prevents the body from metabolizing the amino acid phenylalanine. About 1 in 14,000 babies, or about 300 per year, are born with PKU. Untreated, it leads to mental retardation; a diet low in this one amino acid will allow normal growth and development.

16. U.S. Preventive Task Force, *Guide to Clinical Preventive Services*, (1989), p. xxiii.

17. Council on Scientific Affairs, "Medical evaluation of healthy persons," *JAMA* 249 (1983): 1626–1633.

18. The Canadian action came after numerous meta-evaluations conducted in the 1970s and 1980s, some of which were sponsored by prestigious national or professional organizations, including the American Cancer Society, the American College of Physicians, and the U.S. Preventive Services Task Force.

19. According to one survey of physicians in North Carolina, almost all agreed that primary caregivers should assist asymptomatic patients in reducing behavioral risk factors. Half reported counseling patients who smoke or abuse other drugs; one-fifth counseled patients with diet or nutrition problems. Younger, white female physicians tended to counsel more. See Center for Disease Control, "Effectiveness in disease and injury prevention counseling practices of primary care physicians, North Carolina, 1991." MMWR 41 (1992): 565–568.

20. T. Delbanco, and W. Taylor, "The periodic health examination, 1980," *Annals of Internal Medicine* 92 (1980): 251–252.

21. Christine Lane, "The annual physical examination: needless ritual or necessary routine?" Editorial in *Annals of Internal Medicine* 136 (2002): p. 702.

22. Quoted in Gina Kolata, "Annual physical checkup may be an empty ritua," *New York Times*, August 12, 2003.

23. Agency for Healthcare Research and Quality, "Take a loved one to the doctor day." *Electronic Newsletter*, no. 109, September 12, 2003.

24. The 1996 *Guide* was co-chaired by Robert Lawrence, who held the same position at Harvard as his predecessor, and, as for the 1989 *Guide*, Deputy Assistant Secretary for Health McGinnis. Once again, staff were provided by Health and Human Services.

25. The *Task Force*'s arsenal does not include a failing mark (such grade inflation indicates that *Task Force* members are academics!), suggesting that the panel inevitably avoids the most severe criticisms.

26. Alfred Berg and Janet Allan, "Introducing the New U.S. Preventive Services Task Force," *Guide to Clinical Preventive Services*, Agency for Healthcare Research and Quality, p. M–4.

27. Rina Punglia, et. al., "Effect of verification bias on screening for prostate cancer by measurement of prostate specific antigen," *New England Journal of Medicine* 349 (2003): 335–42.

28. "Editorial, "A fallible prostate cancer test," *New York Times,* July 30, 2003.

29. T. G. Pickering, et. al., "How common is white coat hypertension," *JAMA* 259 (1988): 225–228.

30. There is an important lesson here. Sociologists have long understood that any kind of intervention, even the very act of observing, changes the behaviors of those being studied—a phenomenon called the "Hawthorne Effect." This means that the screening procedure itself—independent of any underlying malaise—may induce some change in the patient's physiology or body chemistry, thus complicating diagnosis.

31. Jennifer Lafata, et. al., "The economic impact of false-positive cancer screens," *Cancer Epidemiology Biomarkers and Prevention* 13 (2004): 2126–32. The Director of screening for the American Cancer Society was critical of the study, especially with the definition of false positives. For colonoscopies, false positives "really return a dividend" because precancerous polyps are removed during the procedure (quoted in "False positives in screening for cancer prove costly, *New York Times*, December 26, 2004). In contemporary political language, this response would be an excellent example of "spinning."

32. In February 2005, the American College of Medical Genetics endorsed screening of all newborns for 29 conditions, a recommendation that has generated considerable controversy over issues of cost, problems with false positives, and especially safety. Over the years, claims one professor of pediatrics, "thousands of normal kids have been killed or gotten brain damage by [routine] screening tests and treatments that turned out to be ineffective or very dangerous." Quoted in Gina Kolata, "Panel to advise testing babies for 29 diseases," *New York Times*, February 25, 2005.

33. Full body computerized tomography (CT scans) is supposed to detect early signs of such diseases as lung and colon cancer, and coronary artery disease. The procedure costs about $1,000, usually not covered by insurance. There is no evidence that it saves lives, but there are high rates of false positives, forcing patients to undergo additional testing. It turns out that a single full-body scan delivers a radiation dose equivalent to about one hundred mammograms, about the same dose received from atomic bomb survivors a mile and a half from the burst site. It is believed that "tens of thousands or conceivably hundreds of thousands" of Americans have the procedure per annum (Editorial, "Reckless full-body medical scans," *New York Times*, September 6, 2004. The editorial is based on D. Brenner and C. Elliston, "Estimated radiation risks potentially associated with full-body CT screening," *Radiology* 232 (2004): 735–8.

34. Caryn Lerman, et. al., "Psychological and behavioral implications of abnormal mammograms," *Annals of Internal Medicine* 114 (1991): 657–661.

35. Salvatore Mangione and Linda Neiman, "Cardiac auscultatory skills of internal medicine and family practice trainees," *JAMA* 278 (1997): 717–722.

36. William Goodson and Dan Moore, "Causes of physician delay in the diagnosis of breast cancer, *Archives of Internal Medicine* 162 (2002): 1343–1348.

37. "Mammogram reading in U.S. is found to trail that in Britain," *New York Times,* October 22, 2003.

38. D. Murray, et al., "Systematic risk factor screening and education: a community-wide approach to the prevention of coronary heart disease," *Preventive Medicine* 15 (1986): 661–672.

39. R. Collins, et. al., "Blood pressure, stroke and coronary heart disease: short-term reductions in blood pressure," *Lancet* 335 (1990): 827–838.

40. See Amnon Sonnenberg, et. al., "Cost-effectiveness of colonoscopy in screening for colorectal cancer," *Annals of Internal Medicine* 133 (2000): 573–584; and Michael Pignone, et. al., "Cost-effectiveness analysis of colorectal cancer screening: A systematic review for the U.S. Preventive Services Task Force," *Annals of Internal Medicine* 137 (2002): 96–104.

Cost-effectiveness is defined as the amount of money spent per estimated year of life extension from a given intervention. As such, both inexpensive and expensive techniques may be cost-effective or ineffective. At times in this book (twice so far) we use this term. Yet we will not use its logic as a primary determinant of our assessments. Common sense mandates that public policy must consider cost. Nonetheless the country is not—at least not yet, we hope—a business enterprise, and thus, our political decisions must have more breadth than price alone. For a discussion particularly relevant to this chapter, see Richard Deyo, "Cost-effectiveness of primary care," *Journal of the American Board of Family Practice* 13 (2000): 47–54. For a summary of the voluminous literature on this subject, see M. Gold, et. al., *Cost Effectiveness in Health and Medicine* (New York: Oxford University Press, 1996).

41. R. Etzioni, et. al., "Over-diagnosis due to prostate specific antigen screening," *Journal of the National Cancer Institute* 94 (2002): 981–990.

42. W. Whittman, "Natural history of low-stage prostate cancer and the impact of early detection," *Urological Clinical Studies North America* 17 (1990): 689–697.

43. David Thomas, et. al., "Randomized trial of breast self-examination in Shanghai: final results," *Journal of the National Cancer Institute* 94 (2002): 1445–1457.

44. R. Harris and L. Kissinger. "Routinely teaching breast self-examination is dead. What does this mean?" *Journal of the National Cancer Institute* 94 (2002): 1420–1421.

45. Quoted in Mary Duenwald, "Putting screening to the test," *New York Times,* October 15, 2002

46. Anthony Miller, et. al., "The Canadian national breast screening study–1: Breast cancer mortality after 11 to 16 years of follow-up." *Annals of Internal Medicine* 137 (2002): 305–315.

47. Harold Sox. "Editorial: Screening mammography for younger women: Back to basics," *Annals of Internal Medicine* 137 (2002): 362.

48. Steven Goodman, "Editorial: The mammography dilemma: A crisis for evidence-based medicine?" *Annals of Internal Medicine* 137 (2002): 364.

49. U.S. Preventive Services Task Force, "Screening for breast cancer: Recommendations and rationale," *Annals of Internal Medicine* 137 (2002):344–346.

50. Not all screening procedures have as their goal the reduction of mortality or morbidity. In 1989, half of all mothers who had live births received ultrasonography in pregnancy. By the turn of the millennium, this procedure had become a routine screening. Ultrasonography is useful in determining the exact date of conception—90% of patients deliver within two weeks of the due date determined by second trimester ultrasound, and in determining multiple gestations which are missed in a third of all cases of clinical examination. The risks of the procedure are minimal. Even so, the 1996 *Task Force* concluded: "Neither early, late, nor serial ultrasound in normal pregnancy has been proven to improve perinatal morbidity or mortality." For routine screening, its recommendation was a "D" for third trimester, and a "C" for first and second trimester.

In the face of this official finding, how do we reconcile the increasing popularity of ultrasonography? Presumably, there is some benefit to the procedure. And there is, but it is one that the *Task Force* does not mention, for it is deemed not to be a medical advantage. Most pregnant women desire ultrasonography to determine the sex of their unborn fetus. One study of a military hospital found that 98% of pregnant women wanted an ultrasonogram. Indeed, more than one-third were willing to pay for the procedure themselves. The first listed reason for the test was "to determine the sex of the fetus," M. B. Stephens, et. al., "The maternal perspective on prenatal ultrasound," *Journal of Family Practice* 49 (2000): 601–604. Screening for the sex of the fetus might involve more than curiosity. In some underdeveloped countries, ultrasound is used to identify female fetuses for selective abortion.

This procedure has no real medical benefit in that it is not associated with a reduction in morbidity or mortality. What is deemed a worthwhile benefit depends on the eyes of the beholder—who in this case are pregnant women. Here is an important point for our book: that the desirability of a given screening is always subjective, and may involve criteria other than mortality and morbidity, and may invoke values that are outside the traditional medical model.

51. American College of Physicians, *The Impending Collapse of Primary Care Medicine and Its Implications for the State of the Nation's Health* (Washington, DC: American College of Physicians, 2006).

Chapter 3: Surgery

1. Richard Selzer, *Letters to a Young Doctor* (NY: Simon & Schuster, 1982).

2. Thomas Pasko and B. Seidman, eds., *Physician Characteristics and Distribution in the United States: 2000–2001 Edition* (Chicago: American Medical Association, 2003).

3. (Ashford, CN: Allied Physicians, Inc., updated, 2002).

4. S. Collins, "Frequency of Surgical procedures among 9000 families," *Public Health Reports* 53 (1938): 1593. Throughout most of the twentieth-century, we knew very little about the frequency and types of surgical procedures in the United States. Now we do. In 1965, the National Center for Health Statistics, through its National Hospital Discharge Survey, began to collect information on the number of inpatient operations performed annually in the United States. The Center for Disease Control's annual National Hospital Ambulatory Medical Care Survey, begun in 1992, gives us detailed information about outpatient surgery.

5. Inexplicably, the 1.4 million abortions per annum are not reported in these outpatient statistics.

6. Data on surgery are from the Center for Disease Control, *National Hospital Discharge Survey of Ambulatory Surgery: 2000 Annual Summary*. National Center for Health Statistics (Washington, DC: U.S. Government Printing Office, 2001).

7. E. Shearer, "Cesarean section: Medical costs and benefits," *Social Science and Medicine* 37 (1993): 1251–60.

8. A Tussing and Martha Worrowycz, "The effect of physician characteristics on clinical behavior: Cesarean section in New York State," *Social Science and Medicine* 37 (1993): 1251–60.

9. S. Koroukian, "Estimating the proportion of unnecessary Cesarean sections in Ohio using birth certificate data," *Journal of Clinical Epidemiology* 51 (1998): 1327–1334.

10. Colin Francome and Wendy Savage, "Cesarean sections in Britain and the United States," *Social Science and Medicine* 37 (1993): 1199–1218.

11. Carol Sakala, "Medically unnecessary Cesarean section births: Introduction to a symposium," *Social Science and Medicine* 37 (1993): 1177–98.

12. *Research Activities*, Agency for Healthcare Research and Quality, October 2003, p. 7.

13. N. Lee, et. al., "Confirmation of pre-operative diagnosis for hysterectomy." *American Journal of Obstetrics and Gynecology* 150 (1984): 283–87.

14. D. Leaque, "Endometrial ablation as an alternative to hysterectomy," *AORN Journal* 77 (2003): 322–38.

15. In another example of what sociologists call the "Hawthorne" effect, one study showed that bureaucratic oversight, decreased the number of hysterectomies by 24%. See J. Gambone, R. Recter and S. Hagey, "The impact of quality assurance process on the frequency and confirmation rate of hysterectomy, *American Journal of Obstetrics and Gynecology* 163 (1990): 545–50."

16. J. Schaffer and A. Word, "Hysterectomy—still a useful operation," *New England Journal of Medicine* 347 (2002): 1360–62.

17. J. Maier and J. Maloni, "Nurse advocacy for selective versus routine episiotomy," *Journal of Obstetric, Gynecologic and Neonatal Nursing* 26 (1997): 155–61.

18. Alice Jacobs, "Coronary stents: have they fulfilled their promise?" *New England Journal of Medicine* 341 (1999): 2005–6.

19. Jassim Al Suwaidi, et. al., "Coronary artery stents," *JAMA*: 248 (2000): 1828–1836.

20. Richard Lange and L. David Hollis, "Use and overuse of angiography and revascularization for acute coronary syndromes," *New England Journal of Medicine* 338 (1998): 1838–9.

21. J. J. Goy, "Intracoronary stenting," *Lancet* 351 (1998): 1943–9.

22. "CASS Principal Investigators and their associates, "Myocardial infarction and mortality in the coronary artery surgery study (CASS) randomized trial," *New England Journal of Medicine* 370 (19984): 750–58.

23. "Bernard Chaitman, et. al., "Myocardial infarction and cardiac mortality in the bypass angioplasty revasculariztion investigation (BARI) randomized trials," *Circulation* 96 (1997): 2162–70.

24. Lange and Hollis, "Use and overuse of angiography," p. 1839.

25. Quoted in Gina Kolata, "New studies cast doubt on artery-opening operations," *New York Times*, March 21, 2004.

26. *New York Times*, "The limits of opening arteries," *New York Times*, March 28, 2004.

27. "L. Cobb, et. al., "An evaluation of internal mammary artery ligation by a double blind technique," *New England Journal of Medicine* 260 (1959): 1115.

28. J. Mosely, et. al., "A controlled trial of arthroscopic surgery for osteoarthritis of the knee," *New England Journal of Medicine* 347 (2002): 81–88.

In another example of sham surgery for Parkinson's Disease, patients had holes drilled into their head but the dura was not penetrated. See Curt Freed, et. al., "Transplantation of embryonic dopamine neurons for severe Parkinson's Disease, *New England Journal of Medicine* 344 (2001): 710–19. Oddly, the study received little attention—positive or negative—we would suppose, because the "real surgery" failed, that is, it showed little effectiveness. One critic's response (C. Weijer, *Journal of Law and Medical Ethics* 30 (2002): 69) to this neurological sham surgery was an article with a title that said it all: "I need a placebo like I need a hole in the head."

29. Though it was lower in clinical two trials (0.1 and 0.6%), presumably because of careful case selection and surgical skill. See Executive Committee for the Asymptomatic Carotid Atherosclerosis Study. "Endarterectomy for asymptomatic carotid artery stenosis," *JAMA* 273 (1995): 1421–28.

NOTES TO CHAPTER 3

Interestingly, small area analysis among Medicare patients showed great variance (from 20 to 110 per thousand) across 306 geographically discreet populations, a variance that was highly correlated to the use of ultrasonography, the diagnostic test for atherosclerosis. John Wennberg and M. Cooper, (eds.) "In other words, the availability and use of the diagnostic procedure dramatically increases the odds of surgery," *The Quality of Medical Care in the United States: A Report on the Medicare Program* (Chicago: American Hospital Publishing, 1999).

30. Marc Mayberg and Richard Winn, "Endarterectomy for asymptomatic carotid artery stenosis," *JAMA* 273: (1995): 1461 1995, Emphasis added.

31. J. Escarce, et. al., "Falling cholecystectomy thresholds since the introduction of laparoscopic cholecystectomy," *JAMA* 273 (1995): 1581–85.

32. David Ransohoff and Charles McSherry, "Why are cholecystectomy rates increasing: An editorial," *JAMA* 273 (1995): 1621–22.

33. David Wennberg, et. al., "Pounds of prevention for ounces of cure: Surgery as a preventive strategy," *Lancet* 353 (1999): S9–S11.

34. N. Kauff, et. al., "Risk-reducing salpingo-oophorectomy in carriers of BRCA1 or BRCA2 mutations," *New England Journal of Medicine* 346 (2002): 1609–15; and T. Rebbeck, et. al., "Prophylactic oophorectomy in carriers of BRCA1 or BRCA2 mutations," *New England Journal of Medicine* 346 (2002): 1616–22.

35. Daniel Haber, "Prophylactic oophorectomy to reduce the risk of ovarian breast cancer in carriers of BRCA mutations," *New England Journal of Medicine* 346 (2002): 1660–63.

36. In a 1922 editorial, "The Unnecessary Operation," the future president of the American College of Surgeons wrote: "There are regrettably some unconscionable pothunters who will operate on anybody that will hold still. Every hospital should eliminate that kind of man." William Haggard, "The unnecessary operation," *Surgical Gynecology and Obstetrics* 35 (1922): 820. In 1946, a physician compared hysterectomies to a "surgical racket." N. Miller, "Hysterectomy: therapeutic necessity or surgical racket?" *American Journal of Obstetrics and Gynecology* 51 (1946): 804–10. "The crime then resembles theft with violence, known technically as robbery," wrote the Secretary of the Council on Professional Practice of the American Hospital Association seven years later. Charles Letourneau, "The legal and moral aspects of 'unnecessary surgery'." *Hospitals* 27 (1953): 82.

37. Angela Holder, "Unnecessary surgery," *JAMA* 213 (1970): 1755–6; "Recent decisions on unnecessary surgery," *JAMA* 222 (1972): 1593–4; "Unnecessary surgery." *JAMA* 232 (1975): 1059–60.

38. Ira Rutkow, "Surgical operations and manpower: Can technical proficiency be maintained?" in *Socioeconomics of Surgery*, ed. Ira Rutkow, 3–31, (St. Louis: Mosby, 1989).

39. M. Pauly, "What is unnecessary surgery?" *Milbank Memorial Fund Quarterly* 57 (1979): 95–117.

40. Rand Corporation, "Health Services Utilization Study," Rand Report, 1987.

41. Virginia Sharpe and Alan Faden, *Medical Harm* (Cambridge: Cambridge University Press, 1998), p. 213.

42. John Wennberg, "Small area variations in the practice style factor," in *Socioeconomics of Surgery*, ed. Ira Rutkow, 6–91 (St. Louis: Mosby, 1989).

43. In addition to hysterectomy and C-section, the most commonly cited unnecessary surgeries are cataract replacement, gallstone surgery, lumbar diskectomy, removal of the prostate, and total hip replacement. A few decades ago, tonsillectomies would have been on this list.

44. Council on Scientific Affairs, American Medical Association, "Neonatal circumcision: Report #10." (2000).

45. Mortality from heart transplants. Sharon Hunt, "Current status of cardiac transplantation," *JAMA* 280 (1998): 1692–1698.

46. Robert Wolfe, et. al., "Comparison of mortality in all patients on dialysis, patients on dialysis awaiting transplantation, and recipients of a first cadaveric transplant," *New England Journal of Medicine* 341 (1999): 1725–30; and Lawrence Hunsicker, "Editorial. A survival advantage for renal transplantation," *New England Journal of Medicine* 341 (1999): 1762–3.

Chapter 4. Emergency Medicine

1. Meaning that neither the patient nor the physician knows which treatment—experimental agent or placebo—is assigned.

2. Unless otherwise noted, all data on emergency room utilization comes from the "National Hospital Ambulatory Medical Care Survey: 2000 Emergency Department Summary," Department of Health and Human Services, Vital and Health Statistics, Advance Data, April 22, 2002 (#326).

3. For an eloquent and poetic—but never romanticized—description of what happens in emergency rooms, we recommend Frank Huyler's *The Blood of Strangers: Stories from Emergency Medicine* (Berkeley, CA: University of California Press, 1999).

4. Lynne Richardson and Ula Hwang, "Access to care: A review of the emergency medicine literature," *Academic Emergency Medicine* 8 (2001): 1030–36.

5. Indeed about 15% of all emergency visits are paid for by Medicare and about 18% by Medicaid. About 15% of all visits were paid for in their entirety (not copayments or paying deductibles) by the patient. This figure is probably an underestimate because many states mandate that emergency departments not bill those without insurance. The National Center for Health Care Statistics

estimates that there were 1.2 million "no charge" visits in 1996. Wesley Fields, et. al., "The Emergency Medical Treatment and Labor Act as a federal health care safety net program," *Academic Emergency Medicine* 8 (2001): 1064–69.

6. Yet contrary to the popular belief that uninsured people are the major cause of increased emergency use, insured Americans accounted for most of the 16% increase in use between 1996 and 2001. P. Cunningham and J. May, "Insured Americans drive surge in emergency department visits," *Center for Studying Health System Change*, October (2003): 70.

7. Another piece of the "appropriateness" puzzle might be mode of transportation. Three-quarters of all patients were "walk-ins," that is, they arrived via their own transportation—whereas 15% came by ambulance and another 2% were brought by police or social services.

8. U.S. General Accounting Office, "Emergency departments: Unevenly affected by growth and change in patient use," No. B–251319 (Washington, DC: Government Printing Office, 1993).

A 1992 study by the National Center for Health Statistics concluded that 55% of all emergency visits were nonurgent, defined as "those made by patients who did not require immediate attention or attention within a few hours," National Hospital Ambulatory Medical Care Survey: 1992 Emergency Department Summary. Department of Health and Human Services, Vital and Health Statistics, Advance Data, 245 (1994): 1–12.

According to a 1994 study, the proportion of nonurgent visits varied widely—from 23% to 37%— from hospital to hospital. (G. P. Young, et. al., "Ambulatory visits to hospital emergency departments. Patterns and reasons for use: 24 hours in the ED study group," *JAMA* 276 (1996): 460–65.

9. National Hospital Ambulatory Medical Care Survey: 2001, Emergency Department Summary. Department of Health and Human Services, Vital and Health Statistics, Advance Data, 321, 2003.

10. Because the emergency department must function 24 hours per day, seven days per week, it has high fixed costs for medical staff, ancillary services, supplies, overhead and administration; at the same time it has low marginal costs—e.g., the cost of one additional visit. Furthermore, redirecting nonurgent visits to other venues would require that such settings be similarly equipped and staffed. P. H. Himmelstein, et. al., "U.S. emergency department costs: no emergency," *American Journal of Public Health* 86 (1996): 1527–31.

11. R. Williams, "The costs of visits to emergency departments," *New England Journal of Medicine* 334 (1996): 642–6.

12. E. Olson, "No room at the inn: A snapshot of an American emergency room," *Stanford Law Review* 46 (1999): 449–501.

13. Rinaldo Bellomo, et. al., "A prospective before-and-after trial of a medical emergency team," *Medical Journal of Australia* 179 (2003): 283: 287.

14. Graham Nichols, et. al., "A cumulative meta-analysis of the effectiveness of defibrillator-capable emergency medical services for victims of out-of-hospital cardiac arrest," *Annals of Emergency Medicine* 34 (1999): 517–25.

What we mean by "meta-analysis" is the systematic location, retrieval, review, and summarization of prior studies. Unlike traditional reviews, meta-analysis involves original research, combining data from different studies through the use of (or creation of) a common index, thereby providing an estimate of the magnitude and statistical significance of the combined treatment effect. Therefore, meta-analysis seeks a single answer from a series of different research studies. See David Cordray and Robert Fisher, "Synthesizing evaluation findings," Pp. 198-231, *The Handbook of Practical Program Analysis*, eds. Joseph Wholey, et al., (San Francisco: Jossey Bass, 1994).

15. Mickey Eisenberg, et. al., "Cardiac resuscitation in the community: The importance of rapid delivery of care and implications for program planning," *JAMA* 241 (1979): 1905–07.

16. Thomas Rea, et. al., "Emergency medical services and mortality from heart disease: A community study," *Annals of Emergency Medicine* 41 (2003): 494–99.

17. I. G. Stiell, et. al., "Improved out-of-hospital cardiac survival through the inexpensive optimization of an existing defibrillation program: OPALS Study Phase II, " *JAMA* 281 (1999): 1175–81.

18. Jeremy Brown and Arthur Kellermann, "The shocking truth about defibrillators," *JAMA* 284 (2000): 1438–41.

19. J. Fedoruk, et. al., "Rapid on-site defibrillation versus community program," *Prehospital and Disaster Medicine* 17 (2002): 102–06. This is an important aside.

The careful reader will have noted that in the casino it took longer to defibrillate (though the equipment was on site), and longer for EMS to arrive, compared with what happened in the previous study of urban and suburban Ontario. Even with these longer times, the casino victims fared better, the opposite of what would be expected. With time being the essence of life versus death, how might we explain this strangeness? We have no answer except this: the more scientific studies one reads, the more inexplicable findings one finds. Any one study should never be the basis of a scientific or policy conclusion

20. Jeremy Brown and Arthur Kellermann, "Shocking truth about defibralators," *JAMA* 284 (2000): 1438–41.

21. J. H. Pope, et. al., "Missed diagnoses of acute cardiac ischemia in the emergency department," *New England Journal of Medicine* 342 (2000): 1163–70. A similar study from Hong Kong found that more than one-quarter of all patients with myocardial infarctions were discharged, principally because of inaccurate electrocardiogram interpretations. W. K. Chan, et. al., "Undiagnosed acute myocardial infarction in the accident and emergency department: reasons and implications," *European Journal of Emergency Medicine* 5 (1998): 219–24.

22. National Institutes of Health, Consensus Statement 46 (1983): 1–26. In 1978, the NIH established the Office of Medical Applications of Research to conduct Consensus Development Conferences which would "hasten the resolution of

scientific issues," especially those with "important social dimensions." Since 1978, there have been several conferences per year. Although some, not unexpectedly, become highly politicized. See G. Markle and D. Chubin, "Consensus development in biomedicine: the liver transplant controversy," *Milbank Quarterly* 65 (1987): 1–24. We applaud the National Institutes of Health for holding these conferences. Problems notwithstanding, CD conferences have contributed both to the public understanding and the scientific conduct of medicine.

23. As with all conferences more than several years old, the CD statement now is tagged with a *caveat*: "This document is no longer viewed by NIH as guidance for current medical practice."

24. Marion Danis, "The survival benefit of intensive care," *Critical Care Medicine* 32, (August 2004).

25. S. Wainwright, et. al., "Cardiovascular mortality—the hidden peril of heat waves," *Prehospital and Disaster Medicine* 14 (1999): 222–31.

26. MMWR, "New York City Department of Health response to terrorist attack, September 11, 2001," *Morbidity and Mortality Weekly Report* 50 (2001): 821–2.

27. Atul Gawande, "Casualties of war—military care for the wounded from Iraq and Afghanistan," *New England Journal of Medicine* 351 (2004): 2471–2475.

Even under primitive conditions, battlefield medicine can be effective. During the battle of Jalalabad, Afghanistan (1989–1992), advanced trauma care prior to hospitalization in rural Pakistan halved the mortality, from 26% to 13%. H. Husum, "Effects of early prehospital life support to war injured: The battle of Jalalabad, Afghanistan," *Prehospital and Disaster Medicine* 14 (1999): 75–80.

28. Todd Taylor, "Threats to the health care safety net," *Academic Emergency Medicine* 8 (2001): 1080–87.

29. A. Harris, et. al., "Murder and medicine: The lethality of criminal assault 1960–1999," *Homicide Studies* 6 (2002): 128–66.

30. R. S. Crampton, "Reduction of pre-hospital, ambulance and community coronary death rates by the community-wide emergency cardiac care system," *The American Journal of Medicine* 58 (1975): 151–65.

31. R. B. Myers, "Pre-hospital management of acute myocardial infarction: Electrocardiogram acquisition and interpretation, and thrombolysis by pre-hospital care providers," *The Canadian Journal of Cardiology* 14 (1998): 1231–40.

32. Thomas Rea, et. al., "Emergency medical services and mortality from heart disease: A community study," *Annals of Emergency Medicine* 41 (2003): 494–99.

33. Rea, "Emergency medical services," p. 494–99.

34. Lars Wik, et. al., "Quality of cardiopulmonary resuscitation during out-of-hospital cardiac arrest," *JAMA* 293 (2005): 299–304.

35. Benjamin Abella, "Quality of cardiopulmonary resuscitation during in-hospital cardiac arrest, *JAMA* 293 (2005): 305–310.

36. Summarized in Arthur Sanders and Gordon Ewy, "Cardiopulmonary resuscitation in the real world: When will the guidelines get the message?" *JAMA* 293 (2005): 363–65.

Chapter 5. Pharmaceuticals

1. Substance Abuse and Mental Health Administration, National Survey on Drug Use and Health, 2004. *Nonmedical Use of Prescription Pain Relievers*, May 21, 2004. (Bethesda, MD: National Institutes of Health). Unless otherwise noted, data which follow are from this survey.

2. Twenty-two percent of young adults (age 18–25) abused pain relievers, about twice as likely as other age groups; males were more likely abusers than females (14% to 11%); whites more likely than blacks (14% to 10%). These data, from the 2003 National Survey on Drug Use and Health, are collected by interviews in which respondents are asked to admit to illegal, or at least questionable, behaviors. For any such "self-reported" data, an unknown proportion of respondents will not tell the truth, fearing embarrassment or self-incrimination. Thus, these data of drug abuse are almost surely underestimates.

3. A search of Lexus-Nexus provides myriad examples. At the University of Arizona Campus Health Center, students have been given prescriptions of Vicodin for sore throats. "I was really surprised," said one student. "I totally expected antibiotics, and all I got was Vicodin. It seems really weird to me. Why are they treating sore throats with these medications?" *Arizona Daily Wildcat*, March 5, 2004.

4. Brian Strom, "Statins and over-the-counter availability," *New England Journal of Medicine* 352 (2005):1403–05.

5. These data come from IMS Health, a company that tracks the pharmaceutical industry. See James Gorman, "The altered human is already here," *New York Times*, April 6, 2004.

6. Americans are taking more drugs. . . . Agency for Healthcare Research and Quality, MEPS, Statistical Brief #56, National Health Care Expenses in the U.S. Community Population, 2001.

7. Robert Pear, "Americans relying more on prescription drugs, report says," *New York Times*, December 3, 2004.

8. Marcia Angell, *The Truth About Drug Companies* (New York: Random House, 2004). Later in the chapter, we will return to the writings of Dr. Angell, who is former editor of the *New England Journal of Medicine*.

9. As of 2005, there were six brands: Lipitor (Pfizer), Zocor (Merck), Crestor (AstraZeneca), Pravachol (Bristol Myers Squibb), Lescol (Reliant), and Mevacor (also by Merck).

10. David Tuller, "Seeking a fuller picture of statins," *New York Times*, July 20, 2004.

11. PROSPER (Prospective Study of Pravastatin in the Elderly at Risk), ALHAT (Antihypertensive and Lipid-Lowering Treatment to Prevent Heart Attack Trial), and ASCOT (Anglo-Scandinavian Cardiac Outcomes Trial). Each was randomized double-blinded; populations ranged from age 55 to 75.

12. M. Vrecer, et. al., "Use of statins in primary and secondary prevention of coronary heart disease and ischemic strokes: Meta-analysis of randomized trials," *International Journal of Clinical Pharmacology and Therapeutics* 41 (2003): 567–77.

13. M. Briel, et. al., "Effects of statins on stroke prevention in patients with and without coronary heart disease: A meta-analysis of randomized controlled trials," *American Journal of Medicine* 117 (2004): 596–606.

14. Therapeutics Initiative, "Do statins have a role in primary prevention?" *Therapeutics Letter* 48 (June, 2003).

15. P. Jackson, et. al., "Statins for primary prevention: At what coronary risk is safety assured?" *British Journal of Clinical Pharmacology and Therapeutics* 52 (2001): 439–46.

16. Bruce Psaty, et. al., "Potential for conflict of interest in the evaluation of suspected adverse drug reactions," *JAMA* 292 (2004): 2622–31. In an invited response, a Bayer attorney accuses the authors of quoting internal company documents "out of context."

17. Quoted in Tuller, "Seeking a fuller picture," p.

18. LIPID (long-term intervention with Prevastatin in ischemic diseases), CARE (cholesterol and recurrent events), and 4S (Scandinavian Simvastatin survival study).

19. B. Cheung, et. al., "Meta-analysis of large randomized controlled trials to evaluate the impact of statins on cardiovascular outcomes," *British Journal of Clinical Pharmacology* 57 (2004): 640–51.

20. Bertram Pitt, "Low density lipoprotein cholesterol in patients with stable heart disease—is it time to shift our goals?" *New England Journal of Medicine*, April 7, 2005.

21. Clinical trials presented in this section used Altace (chemical name, Ramipril). As of 2005, there were 10 other common brands of ACE inhibitors: Accupril, Aceon, Capoten, Lotensin, Mavik, Monopril, Prinivil, Univasc, Vasotec, and Zestril.

22. "Clinical practice and treatment. . . . " Low dose diuretics were also more effective than other "first line treatment strategies"— beta-blockers, calcium channel blockers, alpha-blockers and angiotensin receptor blockers—in preventing cardiovascular problems. Bruce Psaty, et. al., "Health Outcomes associated with various antihypertensive therapies used as first-line agents," *JAMA* 289 (2003): 2534–44.

23. Quoted in Marcia Angell, *The Truth About Drug Companies* (New York: Random House, 2004), p. 97.

24. Heart Outcomes Prevention Evaluation Study Investigators. "Effects of an angiotensin-converting enzyme inhibitor, Ramipril, on cardiovasuclar

events in high-risk patients," *New England Journal of Medicine* 342 (2000): 145–53.

25. M. Flather, et. al., "Long-term ACE-inhibitor therapy in patients with heart failure or left-ventricular dysfunction: a systematic overview of data from individual patients," *Lancet* 355: 1578–81.

26. "There is no evidence that the addition of ACE inhibitors…" PEACE is an acronym for Prevention of Events with Angiotensin Converting Enzyme Inhibition. E. Braunwald, et. al., "Angiotensin-converting enzyme inhibition in stable coronary artery disease," *New England Journal of Medicine* 351 (2004): 2058–68.

27. K. Ueshima, et. al., "Is angiotensin-converting enzyme inhibitor useful in a Japanese population for secondary prevention after acute myocardial infarction? A final report of the Japanese Acute Myocardial Infarction Prospective (JAMP) study," *American Heart Journal* 148 (2004): e8.

28. Yearly costs per death prevented were calculated: ACE inhibitors; 6944 Euros; statins, 20,423 Euros; and aspirin, 1019 Euros. The lesson is obvious, that of these three treatment modalities, aspirin is the most cost-effective. Richard Heller, et. al., "Implementing guidelines in primary care: can population impact measures help?" *BMC Public Health* 3 (2003): 1–7.

29. Frances McCrea, "The Politics of Menopause: The 'Discovery' of a Deficiency Disease," *Social Problems*, 31, no. 1 (1993): 11–123. All quotes in this section are from this paper. Using the same scientific and medical data, British scientists and physicians defined and treated Menopause quite differently, a phenomenon that calls into question the very objectivity of medical science. See Frances McCrea and Gerald Markle, "The Estrogen Replacement Controversy in the United States and Great Britain: Different Answers to the Same Question?" *Social Studies of Science* 14, no. 1 (1984):1–6.

30. N. Keating, et. al., "Use of hormone replacement therapy by post-menopausal women in the United States." *Annals of Internal Medicine* 130 (1999): 545–53.

31. Heidi Nelson, et. al., "Postmenopausal hormone replacement therapy for the primary prevention of chronic conditions: a summary of evidence for the U.S. Preventive Task Force. Agency for Health Care Research and Quality, 2002.

32. The Women's Health Initiative. "Risks and benefits of estrogen plus progestin in healthy menopausal women: Principal results from the Women's Health Initiative randomized controlled trial, *JAMA* 288 (2002): 321–22; R. Chiebowski, et. al., "Influence of estrogen plus progestin on breast cancer and mammography in healthy postmenopausal women: The Women's Health Initiative randomized trial," *JAMA* 289 (2003): 2673–84.

33. S. Shumaker, et. al., "Estrogen plus progestin and the incidence of dementia and mild cognitive impairment in postmenopausal women: the Women's Health Initiative Memory Study: a randomized controlled trial," *JAMA* 289 (2003): 2651–62.

34. Quoted in Denise Grady, "Study finds new risk in hormone therapy," *New York Times*, July 25, 2003.

35. National Institutes of Health, "NIH halts use of COX-2 inhibitor in large cancer prevention trial," Public Release, December 24, 2004.

36. In 2004, Merck spent an estimated $100 million advertising Vioxx. In the first nine months of 2004, Pfizer spent $71.2 million on Celebrex, a 55% increase from the same period in the previous year. Barry Meier, "Medicine fueled by marketing intensified trouble for pain pills," *New York Times*, December 19, 2004.

37. Quoted in Merrill Goozner, *The $800 Million Dollar Pill* (Berkeley, CA: University of California Press, 2004), p. 225.

38. Head of Cardiology at the Cleveland Clinic, Eric Topol, would become a key figure in the controversy over Vioxx, but not without embarrassment to him. In December 2004, *Fortune Magazine* reported that he was a paid consultant for a hedge fund that had made money betting that Merck stock would decline—which his actions helped to cause. In response, Topol ended his relationship with the fund, as well as paid consultancies with Eli Lily, Bristol-Meyers and at least a half dozen other companies. Andrew Pollack, "Medical researcher moves to sever ties to companies," *New York Times*, January 25, 2005.

39. D. Mukherjee, et. al., "Risk of cardiovascular events associated with selective COX-2 inhibitors," *JAMA* 286 (2001): 954–9.

40. Peter Juni, et. al., "Risk of cardiovascular events and rofecoxib: Cumulative meta-analysis," *Lancet* 364 (2004): 2021–29.

41. A. Matthew and B. Martinez, "E-mails suggest Merck knew Vioxx's dangers at early stage," *Wall Street Journal*, November 1, 2004, p. A–1.

42. Alex Berenson and Gardiner Harris, "Pfizer says 1999 trial revealed risks with Celebrex," *New York Times*, February 1, 2005.

43. Richard Horton, "Vioxx, the implosion of Merck, and aftershocks at the FDA," *Lancet* 364 (2004): 1995–6. Merck responded angrily in a letter, dutifully published in *Lancet*. "We believe that to print a comment in a scientific journal, criticizing Merck's ethical standards on the basis of unfounded allegations printed in the lay press, without even the pretense of investigation into their accuracy or completeness, is inappropriate." Peter Kim and Alise Reicin, "Discontinuation of Vioxx," *Lancet* 365 (2005): 23.

44. Quoted in Gardiner Harris, "Study says drug's dangers were apparent years ago," *New York Times*, November 5, 2004.

45. Eric Topol, "Failing the public health—Rofecoxib, Merck, and the FDA," *New England Journal of Medicine* 351 (2004): 1707–09.

46. Eric Topol, "Good Riddance to a bad drug," *New York Times*, October 2, 2004.

47. Ten members of the panel admitted to previous financial ties with either Merck or Pfizer. Nine of those ten voted in favor of Vioxx. These panelists denied that their history influenced their vote in any way. But one physi-

cian complained: "Fifty patients a day probably die from these drugs, and who is speaking for them?" Quoted in Gardiner Harris and Alex Berenson, "10 voters on panel packing pain pills had industry ties," *New York Times*, February 25, 2005.

48. Quoted in Gardiner Harris, "FDA is advised to let pain pills stay on the market," *New York Times*, February 19, 2005.

49. J. Matheson and D. Figgit, "Rofecoxib: A review of its use in the management of osteoarthritis, acute pain and rheumatoid arthritis," *Drugs* 61 (2001): 833–65.

50. Arnold Relman and Marcia Angell, "America's other drug problem," *New Republic*, December 16, 2002. Prior to Angell, Relman was editor-in-chief of the *New England Journal of Medicine*.

51. Dennis Cauchon, "FDA advisors tied to industry," *USA Today*, September 25, 2000, 1A.

52. Phil Fontanarosa, "Postmarketing surveillance—lack of vigilance, lack of trust," *JAMA* 292 (2004): 2647–50.

53. See Gardiner Harris, "Drug makers are still giving gifts to doctors, FDA official says," *New York Times*, March 4, 2005.

Chapter 6: Mental Illness

1. Quoted Glen Gabbard, *The Psychology of the Sopranos* (New York, Basic Books, 2004), p. 23. Some, psychiatrists included, would claim that Tony was "evil," defined as those who are "lethal predators . . . psychopathic, sadistic and sane." One psychiatrist has developed what he calls a "depravity scale," which rate the horror of an act by the sum of its grim details. Another has published a twenty-two-level hierarchy of evil behavior. See Benedict Carey, "For the worst of us, the diagnosis may be 'evil,'" *New York Times*, February 8, 2005. We are not convinced that "evil," essentially a religious term, is helpful in fathoming bad behavior. Our own preference for understanding Tony is to pick one of Carmela's choices

2. Including Lorraine Bracco, who plays Jennifer Melfi, Tony's psychiatrist. In 2005, Pfizer produced a television commercial in which Bracco described how her depression was successfully treated with their product, Zoloft—demonstrating that fact does imitate fiction. (Stephanie Saul, "More celebreties finding roles as antidepressant advocates, *New York Times*, March 21, 2005.

3. National Institute of Mental Health, *The Numbers Count: Mental Disorders in America* (Bethesda, MD: 01–4584, 2001). Sociologists understand that the number of suicides will always be underestimated. The cause of death (e.g., a single car accident) may be ambiguous. Moreover, social and religious stigma, as well as concerns about life insurance payments, may result in other causes listed on death certificates.

4. The advantage is that we learn about untreated problems as well as those treated. The disadvantage is that self-reports, particularly of socially problematic behaviors, are surely underestimates.

5. Note that as expected these estimates are lower than those of NIMH. Ronald Kessler, et. al., "Lifetime and 12-month prevalence of *DSM-III-R* psychiatric disorders in the United States: Results from the National Comorbidity Survey," *Archives of General Psychiatry* 51 (1994): 8–19.

6. Ronald Kessler, et. al., "Past-year use of outpatient services for psychiatric problems in the National Comorbidity Survey," *American Journal of Psychiatry* 156 (1999): 115–23.

7. Of all the states, Massachusetts has the most psychiatrists, 31 per 100,000, North Dakota the least, 9 per 100,000. After the United States comes Canada and the Netherlands (12 per 100,000), still triple the rate for Britain (4 per 100,000). G. Andrews, "Private and public psychiatry: a comparison of health care systems," *American Journal of Psychiatry* 146 (1989): 881–86.

8. Behind internal medicine, family medicine, and pediatrics. In this chapter, we consider only psychiatrists, and do not consider "licensed psychologists," who have a Ph.D. degree. Typically, their practice would be similar to that of a psychiatrist with one important exception: they cannot prescribe medicine, though in recent years some states have allowed psychologists to do just that. Nor are we considering "limited license" practitioners, professionals with various post-baccalaureate degrees in such areas as psychology, social work, and counseling. Most practitioners with limited licenses treat patients with some sort of cognitive therapy.

9. Pasko and Seidman, Physician characterristics, p.

10. James Scully and Joshua Wilk, "Selected characteristics and data of psychiatrists in the United States, 2001–2002," *Academic Psychiatry* 27 (2003): 247–51. The fastest growing psychiatric subspecialty, about 15% of the total, is "child psychiatry,"(which we assume is not psychiatry practiced by children—a frightening thought—and therefore should be called "psychiatry of or for children"). In the past three decades, it grew by 194%.

11. Deborah Zarin, et. al., "Characterizing psychiatry with findings from the 1996 National Survey of Psychiatric Practice," *American Journal of Psychiatry* 115 (1998): 397–404. The data were collected by mail questionnaire, the response to which was 70%. Unfortunately, the authors gave no data to indicate possible bias introduced by the considerable nonresponse.

12. Harold Pincus, et. al., "Psychiatric patients and treatments in 1997," *Archives of General Psychiatry* 56 (1999): 441–49.

13. Occasionally there is a pathology, as in Alzheimer's Disease, though this instance is only confirmed postmortem. Studies of brain chemistry or anatomy in disorders such as schizophrenia yield correlates at best rather than an unambiguous sign which is present in the diseased, absent in the healthy.

14. Not surprisingly, the concept of "illness" or "disease" is difficult to define. The best we have seen, especially with reference to this argument, is that by disease "we mean a condition that is a bad thing to have...that we consider the afflicted person to be unlucky, and that [the condition] can potentially be medically treated." Rachel Cooper, "What is wrong with *DSM*?" *History of Psychiatry* 15 (2004): 5–25.

15. APA, *DSM-III*. (Washington, D.C.: APA, 1980), p. 6.

16. A 5th edition of *DSM* is planned for 2010.

17. APA, *Diagnostic and Statistical Manual-IV*, 4th ed. (Washington, D.C.: APA, 1994), p. xix.

18. Note that the commonly used abbreviation, *DSM*, leaves off the last three words of the actual title, which are:...*of Mental Disorders*. Thus, the APA's title refers to "disorders," not "diseases." The distinction is important. "There could arguably not be a worse term than *mental disorder*," according to the Chair of the *DSM-IV* Task Force, "to describe the conditions classified" in the manual." A. Frances, "Foreword," in *Philosophical Perspectives on Psychiatric Diagnostic Classification*, eds. J. Sadler, et. al., (Baltimore: Johns Hopkins University Press, 1994), p. ix. If disease is difficult to define, disorder is even more problematic. "The term, *mental disorders*," write the authors of the DSM, "unfortunately implies a distinction between 'mental' disorder and 'physical' disorder that is a reductionistic anachronism of mind-body dualism"(APA, p. xxiii).

19. Thomas Szasz, *Pharmacy* (Westport, CT: Praeger, 2004), p. 36, p. 80. The brilliant and intrepid Szasz has been writing about these issues for several decades. Our views of mental illness and mental health have been influenced by his writings, especially his book, *The Myth of Mental Illness*, written in 1961.

20. Arthur Houts, "Discovery, invention, and the expansion of the modern *Diagnostic and Statistical Manuals of Mental Disorders*, in *Rethinking the DSM*, eds. L Beutler and Mary Malik (Washington, DC: American Psychological Association, 2002). We should point out (and applaud the fact that) that this volume was published by the APA, the very organization that created and continues to sponsor the *DSM*.

21. Szas, *Pharmacy*, p. 80

22. Houts, *Mental Disorders*, pp. 48, 50.

23. Quoted in Szasz, *Pharmacy*, p. 27.

24. APA, "Position paper on homosexuality and civil rights," *American Journal of Psychiatry* 131 (1973): 497.

25. National Institutes of Mental Health, *Depression* (Bethesda, MD: #02–3561, 2002).

26. For an analytical but critical history of antidepressants, see two books by David Healy, *The Antidepressant Era* (Cambridge, MA: Harvard University Press, 1997); and *Let Them Eat Prozac* (New York: New York University Press,

2004). Dr. Healy is a Reader in Psychological Medicine at the University of Wales College of Medicine and Director of the North Wales Department of Psychological Medicine.

27. Using the scientific method to evaluate any talking therapy is difficult. First, one can hardly imagine a control group that receives some fake or placebo therapy (empty words?) which is then compared with an experimental group. What can be done is to offer one group a special treatment, while the other receives some baseline "usual" treatment. Thus, so-called blinding let alone double-blinding (even the psychiatrist doesn't know who gets treatment?) is absurd. Second, the very measurement of progress, problematic in any clinical trial, is based not on an objective sign, but rather a symptom which can only be assessed by the patient. Thus, we have a significant "Hawthorne Effect." Since the patient has invested considerable time and energy into the treatment program, he or she is likely to believe in its success. Even more, unlike other medical practice, talking therapy is directly and explicitly dependent on the relationship between patient and physician. Psychoanalysis has a special language to describe the therapeutic opportunities and dangers of this bonding. Measurement, let alone repeated measurement, especially by a third party, would be so intrusive "as to no longer resemble the reality of clinical practice." For a review of this issue, see Stuart Ablon and Enrico Jones, "Validity of controlled clinical trials of psychotherapy: Findings from the NIH treatment of depression collaborative research program," *American Journal of Psychiatry* 159 (2002): 775–83.

28. SSRI stands for Selective Serotonin Reuptake Inhibitors. Our discussion will also include the related SSNI's, Serotonin and Norepinephrine Reuptake Inhibitors. The first SSRI, Prozac, was approved in 1987 for the treatment of depression; the same drug was approved for the treatment of obsessive-compulsive disorder in 1994, for bulimia in 1997, and for geriatric depression in 1999.

29. In 2003, the category, antipsychotic drugs, were fifth in retail dollars.

30. I. Anderson and B. Tomenson, "The efficacy of selective selective serotonin reuptake inhibitors in depression: a meta-analysis of studies against tricyclic antidepressants," *Journal of Psychopharmacology* 8 (1994): 238–49.

31. Healy, *Antidepressant Era*, p. 38.

32. Quoted in Angell, *Truth about Drug Companies* (2004), p. 112–13. The difference between the groups averaged only 2 points on the 62 point Hamilton scale that is routinely used to measure the severity of depression. This finding is statistically significant, which demonstrates that the differences between the two groups were not due to random variation. Statistical significance is necessary but not sufficient to show clinical importance. In other words, a finding which is statistically significant may have little clinical significance.

33. Ronald Ackerman and John Williams, "Rational treatment for nonmajor depression in primary care," *Journal of General Internal Medicine* 17 (2002): 293–301.

34. Gardiner Harris, "FDA panel urges stronger warning on antidepressants," *New York Times*, September 15, 2004.

35. Shaila Dewan and Barry Meier, "Boy who took antidepressant is convicted of killings," *New York Times*, February 16, 2005. The defense attorney, who was involved in civil litigation against Pfizer, claimed that it was "impossible" to separate his client's guilt from the problems with Zoloft.

36. National Center for Health Statistics. Advance Data # 346, August 26, 2004.

37. The blind use of placebos raises obvious ethical questions, particularly when patients have conditions such as depression that might affect their judgment to make informed choices. C. Elliott, "Caring about risks: Are severely depressed patients competent to consent to research?" *Archives of General Psychiatry* 54 (1997): 113–16. In the TADS design, a parent or guardian gives consent for the adolescent.

38. Treatment for Adolescents with Depression Study (TADS) Team, "Fluoxetine, cognitive-behavioral therapy, and their combination for adolescents with depression," *JAMA* 292 (2004): 807–20, especially p. 819.

39. Richard Glass, "Treatment of adolescents with major depression," *JAMA* 292 (2004): 861–3.

40. David Antonuccio and David Burns, "Adolescents with depression," *JAMA* 292 (2004): 2577. For us, the most interesting data comes from the placebo group, which shows substantial improvement. We'll explore these implications in the next chapter.

41. Jon Jureidini, et al., "TADS study raises concerns," *British Medical Journal* 329 (2004): 1343–44.

42. Andrea Cipriani, et. al., "Suicide, depression, and antidepressants," *British Medical Journal* 330:373–5.

43. Dean Fergusson, et. al., "Association between suicide attempts and selective serotonin reuptake inhibitors: systematic review of randomised controlled trials," *British Medical Journal* 330 (2005): 396–404.

44. National Institute of Mental Health, 2004 *Schizophrenia* (Bethesda, MD: National Institute of Mental Health).

45. David Rosenhan, "On being sane in insane places," *Science* 179 (1973): 250–258. Critics have pointed out that the subjects initial interview was untruthful, and that psychiatrists would not expect untruthful responses from those who admit themselves for treatment.

46. S. Pilling, et. al., "Psychological treatments in schizophrenia: II. Meta-analysis of randomized controlled trials of social skills training and cognitive remediation," *Psychological Medicine* 32 (2002): 783–91.

47. Here we rely on an excellent review of drug treatment for schizophrenia. See Robert Freedman, "Schizophrenia," *New England Journal of Medicine* 349 (2003): 1738–49.

48. Especially noted in an editorial is that many studies have been sponsored by the very pharmaceutical companies whose drugs were being evaluated, "raising concerns about potential sources of bias in experimental design or interpretation of outcomes." David Lewis, "Atypical antipsychotic medications and the treatment of schizophrenia," *British Journal of Psychiatry* 159 (2002): 177–9.

49. K. Wahlbeck, et. al., "Dropout rates in randomized antipsychotic drug trials," *Psychopharmacology* 155 (2001): 230–33.

50. A. Mishara and T. Goldberg, "A meta-analysis and critical review of the effects of conventional neuroleptic treatment on cognition in schizophrenia: Opening a closed book," *Biological Psychiatry* 55 (2004): 1013–22.

51. An acute disease in which the white blood cell count drops to extremely low levels leading to high fever, prostration and severe necrotic ulcerations." See G. Honigfeld, et. al., "Reducing clozapine-related morbidity and mortality," *Journal of Clinical Psychiatry* 59 (1998) [suppl 3]: 3–7.

52. R. Keefe, et. al., "The effects of atypical antipsychotic drugs on neurocognitive impairment in schizophrenia: a review and meta-analysis," *Schizophrenia Bulletin* 25 (1999): 201–22.

53. D. Double, "Rethinking childhood depression," *British Medical Journal* 330 (2005): 418.

54. Ella Mathews, "Response to 'a controversy not far enough'." *British Medical Journal* 329 (2005): 1397. Ms. Mathews is Chair for the Canadian National Ad Hoc Committee on the Protection of the Mentally Ill.

55. Quoted in Angell, *Truth about Drug Companies*, p. 88.

56. Maureen Dowd, "Aloft on Bozoloft," *New York Times*, July 3, 2002.

57. Sami Timimi, "Rethinking childhood depression." *British Medical Journal* 329 (2004): 1394–96.

58. Sami Timimi, "It is more controversial to prescribe anti-depressants than not," *British Medical Journal* 329 (2004): 1397.

59. Gabbard, The Psychology of the Sopranos (New York: Basic Books, 2004), p. 15.

60. Thomas Szasz, *Ideology and Insanity* (Garden City, NY: Anchor Books, 1970), p. 24.

61. Beyond the scope of this chapter is the idea that the label itself, in medicalizing certain (but selective) odd or unusual behaviors, is a key component in the creation the so-called mental illness. See Thomas Scheff, *Being Mentally Ill* (Chicago: Aldine, 1966).

Chapter 7. Mind-Body

1. D. Phillips, et. al., "Psychology and survival," *Lancet* 344 (1993): 1142–45.

2. A. Braithwaite and P. Cooper, "Analgesic effects of branding in treatment of headaches," *British Medical Journal* 282 (1981): 1576–78.

3. Howard Spiro. "Clinical reflections on the placebo phenomenon," in Ann Harrington, *The Placebo Effect* (Cambridge: Harvard University Press, 1999), pp. 37–55.

4. A. DeCraen, et. al., "Placebo effect in the acute treatment of migraine: subcutaneous placebos are better than oral placebos," *Journal of Neurology* 247 (2000): 183–88.

5. J. Turner, et. al., "The importance of placebo effect in pain treatment and research," *JAMA* 271 (1994):1609–14.

6. A. Johnson, "Surgery as placebo," *Lancet* 344 (1994): 114042.

7. Such is the strange world of placebos. In what surely sounds like a laissez faire argument against the protection of human subjects, particularly the use of informed consent (a position contrary to our own): the less the regulation, the greater the placebo effect, ergo, the greater the healing.

8. A. Roberts, et. al., "The power of nonspecific effects in medicine and surgery: implications for biological and psychosocial treatments," *Clinical Psychology Review* 13 (1993): 375–91.

9. Stewart Wolf, "The pharmacology of placebos," *Pharmacological Reviews* 2 (1959): 689–704.

10. Raphael Melmed, *Mind, Body, and Medicine* (New York: Oxford University Press, 2001), p. 130.

11. Penelope Green, et. al., "The powerful placebo: Doubting the doubters." *Advances in Mind-Body Medicine* 17 (2001): 298–307.

12. Quoted in Daniel Moerman and Wayne Jonas, "Deconstructing the placebo effect and finding the meaning response," *Annals of Internal Medicine* 136:471–76. This article is one of the most perceptive reviews written on the subject of placebos.

13. D. Spiegel, "Placebos in practice," *British Medical Journal* 329 (2004): 927–8.

14. Howard Spiro, "Clinical reflections on the placebo phenomenon." As sociologists, we are on familiar ground here. Our colleagues conduct research on this interaction between doctor and patient and find all sorts of problems: that the so-called interaction is mostly one-way, doctor to patient; that the physician treats women differently, and with less respect, than men; that cultural differences between doctor and patient sometimes prevent effective communication; and that even under ideal circumstances, the patient may listen, but not comply, with the doctor's direction. What both sociologists and physicians do not consider is that the nature of this interaction actually affects the disease process.

15. David Morris, "Placebo, pain and belief: A biocultural model." in Ann Harrington "The Placebo Effect (Cambridge, MA: Harvard University Press), p. 189.

16. Moerman and Jonas, "Deconstructing placebo effects."

17. Ibid.

Just as a placebo can cause accidental but unwanted side effects, so can it purposefully cause negative outcomes. This is the so-called nocebo phenomenon (or "toxic placebo" or, in extreme cases, "voodoo death"), defined as the cause of sickness or death by the creation of negative expectations. Thus, a diagnosis of cancer does not directly cause death, but may accelerate its occurrence. For a review, see Robert Hahn. "The nocebo phenomenon: scope and foundations," in Ann Harrington, "Placebo effect," p. 56–76.

18. One could argue the opposite. Between 1997 and 2002, there were five serious books on the subject, plus a book of poetry and a novel—each titled *Placebo Effect*—and an average of 4,000 scholarly papers per annum! Nonetheless, these numbers, which sound impressive, pale in comparison to the amount written on standard specialties. It would be fair to say that there is a new and growing interest in placebos.

19. How blind is double-blind? In one review of 27 studies with more than 13,000 patients, clinicians guessed drug allocations correctly 67% of the time, rather than the 50% guess that randomness should induce; patients were correct 65% of the time. Arthur and Elaine Shapiro, *The Powerful Placebo* (Baltimore, MD: Johns Hopkins University Press, 1997), chap. 11.

20. Ted Kaptchuk, "The placebo effect in alternative medicine: can the performance of a healing effect have clinical significance?" *Annals of Internal Medicine* 136 (2002): 817–25.

21. Harrington, "Placebo effect," p. 8.

22. M. Amanzio, et. al., "Response variability to analgesics: A role for activation of dndogenous opiates," *Pain* 90 (2001): 205–15.

23. Bill Moyers, *Healing and the Mind* (New York: Doubleday, 1993), p. 181.

24. National Center for Complementary and Alternative Medicine, *Mind-Body Medicine: An Overview* (Bethesda, MD: National Institutes of Health, 2004).

25. According to a survey conducted in 1997–98, about 19% of the U.S. adult population use at least one of these five techniques. Of those, 90% had visited a physician in the past year. See P. Wolsko, et. al., "Use of mind-body medical therapies," *Journal of General Internal Medicine* 19 (2004): 43–50.

26. John Astin, et. al., "Mind-body medicine: State of the science, implications for practice," *Journal of the American Board of Family Practice* 16 (2003): 131–147.

27. Kirsi Lillberg, et. al., "Stressful life events and risk of breast cancer in 10,808 women: A cohort study," *American Journal of Epidemiology* 157 (2003): 415–23.

28. Epidemiological designs seek correlates of various social characteristics and behaviors with disease incidence and outcomes. Most are retrospective, meaning that the study begins in the present. Researchers question persons with a particular diagnosis, say breast cancer, about prior conditions (e.g., occupa-

tion) or behaviors (e.g., smoking). If these prior factors show up in greater proportion than in the general population (or some matched sample), they are viewed as possible causes of the current condition. Valuable as they are, such studies must contend with selective or degraded memories.

29. Life events are ones that cause significant change and adjustment in the lives of individuals. Most related to health are negative, such as the death of a spouse, divorce, separation, or getting sent to jail—these four being rated the most stressful according to a widely cited article. (T. Holmes and R. Rahe, "The social readjustment rating scale," *The Journal of Psychomatic Research* 11 (1967): 213–25. Others stressful life events are not necessarily stigmatic, such as marriage or pregnancy.

30. Eva Schernhammer, et. al., "Job stress and breast cancer risk: The nurses health study," *American Journal of Epidemiology* 160 (2004): 1079–86.

31. D. Spiegel, et. al., "Effect of psychosocial treatment on survival of patients with metastatic breast cancer," *Lancet* 2 (1989): 888–91.

32. Spiegel, "Social support: How friends, family, and groups can help," in *Mind Body Medicine*, also Daniel Goleman and Joel Gourin, 342 (Yonkers, NY: Consumer Report Books, 1993).

33. Spiegel's work was featured on Bill Moyers television series and book, *Healing and the Mind*.

34. P. Goodwin, et. al., "The effect of group psychosocial support on survival in metastatic breast cancer," *New England Journal of Medicine* 345 (2001): 1719–26.

35. Pamela Goodwin, "Support groups in breast cancer: When a negative result is positive," *Journal of Clinical Oncology* 22 (2004): 4244–46.

36. D. Spiegel, "Mind matters—group therapy and survival in breast cancer," *New England Journal of Medicine* 345 (2001): 1767–8.

37. D. Spiegel, "Social support: How friends, family, and groups can help," in *Mind Body Medicine*, eds. Daniel Goleman and Joel Gurin, 332–349. (Yonkers, NY: Consumer Report Books, 1993), p. 342.

38. He continues: "... although disentangling the deleterious effects of disease progression on mood complicated this research, as does the fact that some symptoms of cancer and its treatment mimic depression." Spiegel suggests psychophysiological mechanisms, such as deregulation of the hypothalmic-pituitary-adrenal axis, especially diurnal variations in cortisol and melatonin, that might account for this effect. David Spiegel and Janine Griese-Davis, "Depression and cancer: mechanism and disease progression," *Biological Psychiatry* 54 (2003): 269–82.

39. James Goodwin, et. al., "The effects of marital status on stage, treatment, and survival of cancer patients," *JAMA* 258 (1987): 3125–30.

40. A. Neale, et. al., "Marital status, delay in seeking treatment, and survival from breast cancer," *Social Science and Medicine* 23 (1986): 305–312. The authors point unmarried women might have more difficulty than their married

counterparts in seeking diagnosis, keeping appointments, and staying in treatment programs, especially those that are debilitating.

41. Ted Kapchuk, "Powerful placebo: The dark side of the randomized controlled trial," *Lancet* 351(1998): 1722–25.

42. Ann Harrington, "Introduction," in *The Placebo Effect, ed.* Ann Harrington (Cambridge: Harvard University Press, 1999), pp 1–12. This entire collection of articles and essays has been quite helpful to us.

43. Thomas Kuhn, *The Structure of Scientific Revolutions* (Chicago: University of Chicago Press, 1962).

44. George Engel, "The need for a new medical model: A challenge for biomedicine," *Science* 196 (1975): 130, 132.

45. Ibid.

46. Oliver Sacks, *An Anthropologist on Mars* (New York: Alfred A. Knopf, 1995), p. xvi.

Chapter 8. A World Without Medicine

1. McKeown, Role of Medicine p. vii

2. Stephen Bent, et. al., 2006. An accompanying editorial (Robert Paola and Ronald Morton, 2006) claims that this botanical should now be termed an "unproven" method of treatment. Fair enough, as long as the same criterion is applied to any and all conventional medicinals as well.

3. Data are from the 1999–2000 National Health and Nutrition Examination Survey. Use was equal among men and women, higher (23%) for those over 60, for Whites (14% as opposed to 4% for African Americans). See Earl Ford, et. al., "The prevalence of high intake of vitamin E from the use of supplements among U.S. adults," *Annals of Internal Medicine* 143 (2005): 116–20.

4. Almost as many used aspirin. J. Mehta, "Intake of antioxidants among American cardiologists," *American Journal of Cardiology* 79 (1997): 1558–60.

5. The Heart Outcomes Prevention Evaluation Study Investigators, "Vitamin E supplementation and cardiovascular eents in high-risk patients," *New England Journal of Medicine* 342 (2000): 154–160.

6. C. Morris, et. al., "Routine vitamin supplementation to prevent cardiovascular disease: A summary of evidence for the US Preventive Services Task Force," *Annals of Internal Medicine* 239 (2003): 56–70.

7. HOPE and HOPE-TOO Trial Investigators, "Effects of long-term vitamin E supplementation on cardiovascular events and cancer," *JAMA* 293 (2005): 1338–48.

8. B. Greg Brown and John Crowley, "Is there any hope for vitamin E?" *JAMA* 293: 1387–1390.

9. Eliseo Guallar, et. al., "*Annus horribilis* for vitamin E," *Annals of Internal Medicine* 143 (2005): 143–45.

10. Lee, I-Min, et. al., "Vitamin E in the primary prevention of cardiovascular disease and cancer," *JAMA* 294 (2005): 56–65.

11. There are many factors that influence bioavailability. Alice Lichtenstein and Robert Russell, "Essential nutrients: food or supplements?" *JAMA* 294 (2005): 351–58.

12. Catherine MacLean, et. al., "Effects of omega-3 fatty acids on cancer risk," *JAMA* 295 (2006): 403–415.

13. Ross Prentice, et. al., "Low-fat dietary pattern and risk of invasive breast cancer," *JAMA* 295 (2006): 629–42; Shirley Beresford, et. al., "Low fat dietary pattern and risk of colorectal cancer," *JAMA* 295: 643–54; Barbara Howard, et. al., "Low fat dietary pattern and risk of cardiovascular disease," *JAMA* 295 (2006): 655–66.

14. Ali Mokdad, et. al., "Actual cause of death in the United States, 2000," *JAMA* 291 (2004): 1238–45.

15. Center for Disease Control. "Annual smoking-attributable mortality, years of potential life lost, and productivity loses—United States, 1997–2001." *MMWR Weekly* 54 (2005): 625–28.

16. Ibid.

17. J. Barnoya and S. Glantz, "Cardiovascular effects of secondhand smoke: Nearly as large as smoking," *Circulation* 111 (2005): 2684–98.

18. Soon after the code appeared, Philip Morris spent more than $2 million to influence the government process for creating and using medical codes. As of 2004, the code remained "an invalid entry" on common medical forms. Let us not underestimate the political power of the tobacco companies to negatively influence our health policy. See D. Cook, et. al., "The power of paperwork: How Philip Morris neutralized the medical code for secondhand smoke," *Health Affairs* 24 (2005): 994–1004.

19. Allison Hedley, et. al., "Prevalence of overweight and obesity among US children, adolescents, and adults, 1999–2002. *JAMA* 291 (2004): 2847–2850. Weight categories are defined by body-mass index: overweight=BMI 25-25.9; obese=BMI 30–39.0; extreme obesity=BMI 40 or greater.

20. Kenneth Adams, et. al., "Overweight, obesity and mortality in a large prospective cohort of persons 50 to 71 years old," *New England Journal of Medicine* 355 (2006): 763–778.

21. Underweight, the historically more dangerous problem, was responsible for 33,746 excessive deaths. Katherine Flegal, et. al., "Excess deaths associated with underweight, overweight and obesity," *JAMA* 293 (2005): 1861–1867.

22. Heena Santry, et. al., "Trends in bariatric surgical procedures," *JAMA* 294 (2005): 1909–17.

23. Bruce Wolfe and John Morton, "Weighing in on bariatric surgery," *JAMA* 294 (2005): 1960–63.

24. D. Flum, et. al., "Early mortality among medicare beneficiaries undergoing bariatric surgical procedures," *JAMA* 294 (2005): 1903–08.

25. Robert Steinbrook, "Imposing personal responsibility for health," *New England Journal of Medicine* 55 (2006): 753–56.

26. Ronald Troyer and Gerald Markle, *Cigarettes: The Battle Over Smoking* (New Brunswick, NJ: Rutgers University Press, 1983).

27. Center for Disease Control, "State smoking restrictions for private-sector worksites, restaurants, and bars—United States, 1998 and 2004." *MMWR* 54 (2005): 649–653.

28. Richard Sargent, et. al., "Reduced incidence of admissions for myocardial infarction associated with public smoking ban: Before and after study." *British Medical Journal* 328 (2004): 977–980. The lead author was quoted in "Rosemary Ellis, "The secondhand smoking gun," *New York Times*, October 15, 2003.

29. Eric Nagourney, "Doctors use casino as lab to test secondhand smoke," *New York Times*, December 23, 2003.

30. A. Drewnowski and N. Darmon, "The economics of obesity: Dietary energy density and energy cost," *American Journal of Clinical Nutrition* 82 (2005): 265S–273S.

31. Therapeutics Initiative, "Do statins have a role in primary prevention?" *Therapeutics Letter* 48: (June, 2003).

32. By comparison, Japan spends 8% of its GDP, the figure for Germany is 11%. Organization for Economic Cooperation and Development, *OECD Health Data, 2004. A Comparative Analysis of 29 Countries* (Paris: OECD, 2004).

33. Indeed, many underdeveloped countries have more impressive health statistics than the United States. For example, in Albania, an impoverished country with little advanced medical infrastructure or technology, life expectancy is 77.2, just a half year less than ours. U.S. Bureau of the Census, *Infant Mortality and Life Expectancy for Selected Countries, 2005* (Washington, DC: U.S. Government Printing Office, 2005).

34. James Banks, et. al., "Disease and disadvantage in the United States and in England," *JAMA* 295 (2006): 2037–2045. In both countries, there is an "SES gradiant," meaning that poorer people are more sickly than their richer counterparts.

35. National Cancer Institute, *Fact Book*, p. vii. National Institutes of Health, 2004.

36. "Tobacco subsidies in the United States," Farm subsidy database, 2004.

Notes for Appendix A: Alternative Medicine

1. James Reston, "Now let me tell you about my appendectomy in Peking..." *New York Times*, July 26, 1971. As Reston probably understood, the relation between the past and present is neither simple, nor unidirectional.

Fran and I understand all too well that just as the past determines the present, so may the present greatly influence our understanding of the past. See Gerald Markle and Francis B. McCrea, "Forgetting and Remembering: Bitburg and the social construction of history," *Perspectives on Social Problems* 2 (1990): 143–159.

2. By contrast, "mainstream" medicine is also known as "orthodox," "regular," "scientific," "Western," "modern," or especially by its critics, "allopathic." James Dalen, "'Conventional' and 'unconventional' medicine. Can they be integrated?" *Archives of Internal Medicine* 158 (1998): 2179. This article by the editor introduces an entire issue on "Alternative Medicine."

3. E. Ernst, et. al., "Complementary medicine—a definition," *British Journal of General Practice* 45 (1995): 506.

4. David Eisenberg, et. al., "Trends in alternative medicine use in the United States, 1990–1997." *Journal of the American Medical Association* 280 (1998): 1569–1575.

5. James Dalen, "Conventional and unconventional medicine: An editorial." *Archives of Internal Medicine*, Nov 20, 1998.

6. National Institutes of Health Panel Issues Consensus Statement on Acupuncture, NIH News Release, November 5, 1997.

7. Between 1998, some 14% of the population used herbal medicines and other natural products, a proportion that increased to 18% in 2002. There was no change among younger people, but use doubled for those over age 65. Use of *Ginko biloba* and *Panax ginsing* declined, while use of lutein increased dramatically, presumably because of its inclusion in multivitamins. Judith Kelly, et. al., "Recent trends in use of herbal and other natural products," *Archives of Internal Medicine* 165 (2005): 281–86.

8. Eisenberg, "Trends in alternative medicine, 1997.

Notes to Appendix B. Thought Experiments

1. Much of this material is technical. One interesting and readable source is Ian Marshall and Danah Zohar, *Who's Afraid of Schrodinger's Cat* (New York: William Morrow, 1997).

2. Roy Sorensen, *Thought experiments* (New York: Oxford, 1992), p. 7.

3. John Norton, "Thought experiments in Einstein's work," in *Thought Experiments in Science and Philosophy*, eds. Tamara Horowitz and Gerald Massey, 129–144 (Savage, MD: Rowman & Littlefield, 1991), p. 129.

4. Sorensen, *Thought Experiments*, 209–210.

5. Ibid, p. 214.

6. See Marguerite LaCaze, *The Analytic Imagery*. Ithaca (Cornell University Press, 2002); and T. Gendler, *Thought Experiment: On the Power and Limits of Imaginary Cases* (New York: Garland, 2000).

7. Sorensen, *Thought experiments*, p. 17.

8. Kai Erikson. *Everything in its Path: Destruction of Community in the Buffalo Creek Flood* (NY: Simon & Schuster, 1976).

9. Thomas Kuhn. "A function for thought experiments," pp. 240–266 in *The Essential Tension*, ed. Thomas Kuhn, 260–266 (Chicago: University of Chicago Press, 1977)

Notes to Appendix C. Medicine and Mentality

1. Thomas McKeown, "Fertility, mortality and causes of death," *Population Studies* 32 (1978): 535. All mortality data are "age adjusted."

2. Stephen Kunitz, "The personal physician and the decline in mortality," in *The Decline of Mortality in Europe*, eds. R. Schofield, D. Reher and A. Bideau. (Oxford: Clarendon Press, 1991), p. 248.

3. John McKinley, "A case for refocusing upstream," *in Applying Behavioral Science to Cardiovascular Risk* (NY: American Heart Association, (year), p. 144.

4. There were large racial disparities. For whites, the rate was 5.8 per thousand, compared to 13.8 for blacks, 5.6 for Hispanics, and 4.8 for Asians.

5. Richard Meckel, *Save the Babies: American Public Health Reform and the Prevention of Infant Mortality* (Baltimore, MD: Johns Hopkins Press, 1990), p. 1.

6. Robert Anderson, "United States Life Tables," 1998. *National Vital Statistics Report* 48 (#18), February 7, 2001, Table 11. In 1900, a white male could expect another 9.0 years of life; in 1970 he would have an additional year and one-half. White females have gained four years in longevity, from 9.6 in 1900 to 13.6 in 1970. For black males, the improvement has been almost three years, from 8.3 to 11.2; the improvement for black females was almost identical to their white counterparts.

7. Thomas Lewis, *Lives of a Cell*, (New York: Viking, 1974), pp. 34–35. Thomas does acknowledge that "for all this new knowledge, we still have formidable diseases, still unsolved, lacking satisfactory explanation, lacking satisfactory treatment." At the time of his death in 1992, Thomas was CEO of the Sloan-Kettering Institute. Previously, he has been dean of the medical schools at Yale and New York University. He was the author of several widely read books about science and medicine.

8. Evelynn Hammonds, *Childhood's Deadly Scourge: The Campaign to Control Diphtheria in New York City, 1880–1930* (Baltimore, MD: Johns Hopkins Press, 1999), pp. 6–7.

9. Terra Ziporyn, *Diseases in the Popular American Press: The Case of Diphtheria, Typhoid Fever, and Syphilis, 1870–1920* (New York: Greenwood Press, 1988), p. 25.

10. Unless otherwise noted, reference are to John B. McKinley and Sonja M. McKinley, "The questionable contribution of medical measures to the decline in mortality in the United States in the Twentieth Century," *Milbank*

Memorial Fund Quarterly 55 (1977): 405–428; and Thomas McKeown, *The Role of Medicine: Dream, Mirage or Nemesis?* (Princeton, NJ: Princeton University Press, 1979).

11. According to Thomas McKeown, this might be an overestimation, since until 1855 diphtheria was categorized with scarlet fever. In the same year, however, deaths from "croup" were combined with diphtheria, a practice consistent with today's classifications. The name, "diphtheria," was not coined until 1826, but its diagnosis was contested (therefore affecting the quality of mortality data) until the end of the nineteenth century.

12. McKinley, table 1, p. 418. Data from Denmark, Sweden, and Belgium are consistent with these findings. See Marie-France Morel, "The care of children: The influence of medical innovation and the medical institutions on infant mortality, 1750–1914." in R. Schofield, *The Decline of Mortality in Europe* (Oxford: Clarendon Press, 1991). Pp. 196–219.

13. A better case for orthodoxy would be smallpox, where an effective vaccine reduced the death rate to near zero. Yet, smallpox is problematic for orthodoxy, for the vaccine was introduced in 1800, long before the advent of modern medicine.

But the vaccine is not without problems. Prior to the 2003 war in Iraq, the Center for Disease Control recommended against routine smallpox immunization, presumably because the threat of bioterrorism was small, but also because moderate to severe adverse reactions from the vaccine were not uncommon.

14. McKeown, *Role of Medicine*, pp. 92–95. The effectiveness of BCG is in doubt. It was never used systematically in the Netherlands, which nonetheless had by 1969 the lowest death rate from tuberculosis.

15. McKinley, "Fertility, mortality, causes of death," pp. 420–421. These findings are consistent with the histories for water and food-born diseases. In the former, cholera, diarrhea, and dysentery, which were grouped together, had fallen by 95% before the mid-1930s when intravenous treatments became available. For the latter, death from "convulsions and teething," were probably due to whooping cough, measles, and meningitis, most of which had almost disappeared before the advent of vaccines. Most of the decline in so-called noninfectious diseases has come from "prematurity, immaturity, and other diseases of infancy" a category that is no longer used today.

16. McKinley, "Fertility, mortality, causes of death," pp. 424–425. The diseases are tuberculosis, scarlet fever, influenza, pneumonia, diphtheria, whooping cough, measles, smallpox, typhoid, and poliomyelitis. Most of these diseases have been eliminated, or nearly so, in the United States. But the world has become a much smaller place. In 2005, an unvaccinated girl, returning from a visit to Rumania, initiated 34 cases of measles in Indiana. See Amy Parker, et. al., "Implications of a 2005 measles outbreak in Indiana for sustained elimination of measles in the United States," *New England Journal of Medicine* 355 (2006): 447–55.

17. McKinley, "Fertility, mortality, causes of death," p. 406, emphasis in the original.

18. McKeown, *Role of Medicine*, p. 77.

19. Ibid., p. 78.

20. Rene Dubos, *Mirage of Health* (New York: Perennial Library, 1959), p. 23.

Bibliography

Abbasi, Kamran. 2005. "Pills, Thrills, and Bellyaches." *British Medical Journal* 330: 372.

Abella, Benjamin. 2005. "Quality of Cardiopulmonary Resuscitation During In-hospital Cardiac Arrest." *JAMA* 293: 305–310.

Ablon, Stuart and Enrico Jones. 2002. "Validity of Controlled Clinical Trials of Psychotherapy: Findings from the NIH Treatment of Depression Collaborative Research Program." *American Journal of Psychiatry* 159: 775–83.

Ackerman, Ronald and John Williams. 2002. "Rational Treatment for Non-major Depression in Primary Care." *Journal of General Internal Medicine* 17: 293–301.

Adams, Kenneth, et. al., 2006. "Overweight, Obesity and Mortality in a Large Prospective Cohort of Persons 50 to 71 Years Old." *New England Journal of Medicine* 355: 763–778.

Agency for Health Care Research and Quality. 2004. "Prehypertension is a Considerable Health Risk, Particularly in People Aged 45 and Older." *Research Activities*, no. 291, November.

ALLHAT Collaborative Research Group. 2002. "Major Outcomes in Moderately Hypercholesterolemic, Hypertensive Patients Ramdomized to Reavastatin vs Usual Care." *JAMA* 288: 2998–3007.

Alonso, Yolanda. 2004. "The Biopsycosocial Model in Medical Research: The Evolution of the Health Concept over the Last Two Decades." *Patient Education and Counseling* 53: 239–44.

Al Suwaidi, Jassim, et. al., 2000. "Coronary Artery Stents." *JAMA* 248: 1828–1836.

Amanzio, M., et. al. 2001. "Response Variability to Analgesics: A Role for Activation of Endogenous Opiates." *Pain* 90: 205–15.

American College of Physicians. 1991. "Preventive Care Guidelines: 1991." *Annals of Internal Medicine* 114: 758–783.

———. 2006. *The Impending Collapse of Primary Care Medicine and Its Implications for the State of the Nation's Health.* Washington, DC: American College of Physicians.

American College of Surgeons. 1983. "Statement on Unnecessary Surgery." American College of Surgeons' Reports, August.

American Psychiatric Association. 1973. "Position Paper on Homosexuality and Civil Rights." *American Journal of Psychiatry* 131: 497.

———. 1980. *Diagnostic and Statistical Manual-III.* 3rd ed. Washington, DC: APA.

———. 1994. *Diagnostic and Statistical Manual-IV,* 4th ed. Washington, DC: APA.

Anderson, I., and B. Tomenson. 1994. "The Efficacy of Selective Serotonin Reuptake Inhibitors in Depression: a Meta-analysis of Studies Against Tricyclic Antidepressants." *Journal of Psychopharmacology* 8: 238–49.

Anderson, Robert. 2001. "United States Life Tables, *1998.*" *National Vital Statistics Report* 48 (#18).

Andrews, G. 1989. "Private and Public Psychiatry: A Comparison of Health Care Systems." *American Journal of Psychiatry* 146: 881–86.

Angell, Marcia. 2004. *The Truth About Drug Companies.* New York: Random House.

Antonuccio, David, and David Burns. 2004. "Adolescents With Depression." *JAMA* 292: 2577.

Astin, John, et. al. 2003. "Mind-body Medicine: State of the Science, Implications for Practice." *Journal of the American Board of Family Practice* 16: 131–147.

Avanstar Communications. 2004. "A Snapshot of 2003 Market." *Drug Topics* 148 (April 15): 68.

Balas, M., L. Scott, and A. Rogers. 2004. "The Prevalence and Nature of Errors and Near Errors Reported by Hospital Staff Nurses." *Applied Nursing Research* 17: 224–30.

Banks, James, et. al. 2006. "Disease and Disadvantage in the United States and in England." *JAMA* 295: 2037–45.

Barnoya, J., and S. Glantz. 2005. "Cardiovascular Effects of Secondhand Smoke: Nearly as Large as Smoking." *Circulation* 111: 2684–98.

Bellomo, Rinaldo, Trial of a Medical Emergency Team. 2003. "A Prospective Before-and-After." *Journal of Australia* 179: 283, 287.

Bent, Stephen, et. al. 2006. "Saw Palmetto for Benign Prostatic Hyperplasia." *New England Journal of Medicine* 354: 557–66.

Berenson, Alex and Gardiner Harris. "Pfizer Says 1999 Trial Revealed Risks with Celebrex." *New York Times*, February 1, 2005.

Beresford, Shirley, et. al. "Low Fat Dietary Pattern and Risk of Colorectal Cancer." *JAMA* 295: 643–54.

Berg, Alfred and Janet Allan, "Introducing the New U.S. Preventive Services Task Force." In *Guide to Clinical Preventive Services*. Agency for Healthcare Research and Quality, p. M-4.

Blendon, Robert, et. al. 2002. "Views of Practicing Physicians and the Public on Medical Errors." *New England Journal of Medicine* 347: 1933–1940.

Bodenheimer, Thomas. 2006. "Primary Care—Will It Survive?" *New England Journal of Medicine* 355: 861–61.

Braithwaite, A., and P. Cooper. 1981. "Analgesic Effects of Branding in Treatment of Headaches." *British Medical Journal* 282: 1576–78.

Braunwald, E., et. al. "Angiotensin-convertiing Enzyme Inhibition in Stable Coronary Artery Disease." *New England Journal of Medicine* 351: 2058–68.

Brenner, D., and C. Elliston. 2004. "Estimated Radiation Risks Potentially Associated with Full-body CT Screening." *Radiology* 232: 735–8.

Briel, M., et. al. 2004. "Effects of Statins on Stroke Prevention in Patients with and without Coronary Heart Disease: A Meta-analysis of Randomized Controlled Trials." *American Journal of Medicine* 117: 596–606.

Brown, B. Greg and John Crowley. "Is There Any Hope for Vitamin E?" *JAMA* 293: 1387–1390.

Brown, Jeremy, and Arthur Kellermann. 2000. "The Shocking Truth About Defibrillators." *JAMA* 284: 1438–41.

Carey, Benedict. 2005. "For the Worst of Us, the Diagnosis May Be 'Evil'." *New York Times*, February 8.

CASS Principal Investigators and their associates. 1984. "Myocardial Infarction and Mortality in the Coronary Artery Surgery Study (CASS) Randomized Trial." *New England Journal of Medicine* 370: 750–58.

Cauchon, Dennis. 2000. "FDA Advisors Tied to Industry." *USA Today*, September 25, p. 1A.

Center for Disease Control. 1992. "Effectiveness in Disease and Injury Prevention Counseling Practices of Primary Care Physicians, North Carolina, 1991." MMWR 41: 565–568.

————. 1995. National Nosocomial Infections Surveillance. Center for Disease Control.

————. 2001. National Ambulatory Medical Care Survey: 1999 Summary. Center for Disease Control, Vital and Health Statistics 322, July 17.

————. 2005. "Annual Smoking-Attributable Mortality, Years of Potential Life Lost, and Productivity Loses—United States, 1997–2001. *MMWR Weekly* 54: 625–28.

————. 2005. "State Smoking Restrictions for Private-sector Worksites, Restaurants, and Bars—United States, 1998 and 2004." *MMWR* 54: 649–653.

Chaitman, Bernard, et. al. 1997. "Myocardial Infarction and Cardiac Mortality in the Bypass Angioplasty Revasculariztion Investigation (BARI) Randomized Trials." *Circulation*: 96: 2162–70.

Chan, W. K., et. al. 1998. "Undiagnosed Acute Myocardial Infarction in the Accident and Emergency Department: Reasons and Implications." *European Journal of Emergency Medicine* 5: 219–24.

Charap, Mitchell. 1981 "The Periodic Health Examination: Genesis of a Myth." *Annals of Internal Medicine* 95: 733–735.

Cheung, B., et. al. 2004. "Meta-analysis of Large Randomized Controlled Trials to Evaluate the Impact of Statins on Cardiovascular Outcomes." *British Journal of Clinical Pharmacology* 57: 640–51.

Chiebowski, R. T., et. al. 2003. "Influence of Estrogen Plus Progestin on Breast Cancer and Mammography in Healthy Postmenopausal Women: The Women's Health Initiative Randomized Trial." *JAMA* 289: 2673–84.

Cipriani, Andrea, et. al. "Suicide, Depression, and Antidepressants." *British Medical Journal* 330: 373–5.

Cobb, L., et. al. 1959. "An Evaluation of Internal Mammary Artery Ligation by a Double-blind Technique." *New England Journal of Medicine* 260: 1115.

Collins, R., et. al. 1990. "Blood Pressure, Stroke and Coronary Heart Disease: Short-term Reductions in Blood Pressure." *Lancet* 335: 827–838.

Collins, S. 1938. "Frequency of Surgical Procedures Among 9000 Families." *Public Health Reports* 53: 1593.

Cook, D., et. al. 2005. "The Power of Paperwork: How Philip Morris Neutralized the Medical Code for Secondhand Smoke." *Health Affairs* 24: 994–1004.

Cooper, Rachel. 2004. "What is Wrong With *DSM*? *History of Psychiatry* 15: 5–25.

Cordray, David and Robert Fisher. 1994. "Synthesizing Evaluation Findings." Pp. 198-231. In *The Handbook of Practical Program Analysis*, edited by Joseph Wholey, et. al., San Francisco: Jossey Bass.

Council on Scientific Affairs. 1983. "Medical Evaluation of Healthy Persons." *JAMA* 249: 1626–1633.

Crampton, R. S. 1975. "Reduction of Pre-hospital, Ambulance and Community Coronary Death Rates by the Community-wide Emergency Cardiac Care System." *The American Journal of Medicine* 58: 151–65.

Cunningham, P., and J. May. 2003. "Insured Americans Drive Surge in Emergency Department Visits." *Center for Studying Health System Change*, October 70.

Dalen, James. 1998. "'Conventional' and 'Unconventional' Medicine. Can They be Integrated?" *Archives of Internal Medicine* 158: 2179.

Danis, Marion. 2004. "The Survival Benefit of Intensive Care." *Critical Care Medicine* 32, (August).

DeCraen, A., et. al. 2000. "Placebo Effect in the Acute Treatment of Migraine: Subcutaneous Placebos are Better than Oral Placebos." *Journal of Neurology* 247: 183–88.

Delbanco, T., and W. Taylor. 1980. "The Periodic Health Examination, 1980." *Annals of Internal Medicine* 92: 251–252.

Dewan, Shaila and Barry Meier. 2005. "Boy Who Took Antidepressant is Convicted of Killings." *New York Times*, February 16.

Deyo, Richard. 2000. "Cost-effectiveness of Primary Care." *Journal of the American Board of Family Practice* 13: 47–54.

Double, D. 2005. "Rethinking Childhood Depression." *British Medical Journal* 330: 418.

Dowd, Maureen. 2002. "Aloft on Bozoloft." *New York Times*, July 3.

Drewnowski, A., and N. Darmon. 2005. "The Economics of Obesity: Dietary Energy Density and Energy Cost." *American Journal of Clinical Nutrition* 82: 265S–273S.

Dubos, Rene. 1969. *Mirage of Health*. NY: Harper & Row.

———. 1968. *Man, Medicine and Environment*. London: Pall Mall Press.

Duenwald, Mary. 2002. "Putting Screening to the Test," *New York Times*, October 15.

Eisenberg, David, et. al. 1998. "Trends in Alternative Medicine Use in the United States, 1990–1997." *JAMA* 280 no. 11.

Eisenberg, Mickey, et. al. 1979. "Cardiac Resuscitation in the Community: The Importance of Rapid Delivery of Care and Implications for Program Planning." *JAMA* 241: 1905–07.

Elliott, C. 1997. "Caring About Risks: Are Severely Depressed Patients Competent to Consent to Research?" *Archives of General Psychiatry* 54: 113–16.

Ellis, Rosemary. 2003. "The Secondhand Smoking Gun." *New York Times*, October 15.

Engel, George. 1975. "The Need for a New Medical Model: A Challenge for Biomedicine." *Science* 196: 129–136.

Erikson, Kai. 1976. *Everything in its Path: Destruction of Community in the Buffalo Creek Flood*. NY: Simon & Schuster.

Ernst, E., et. al. 1995. "Complementary Medicine—a Definition." *British Journal of General Practice* 45: 506.

Escarce, J., et. al. 1995. "Falling Cholecystectomy Thresholds Since the Introduction of Laparoscopic Cholecystectomy." *JAMA* 273: 1581–85.

Etzioni, R., et. al. 2002. "Over-diagnosis Due to Prostate Specific Antigen Screening." *Journal of the National Cancer Institute* 94: 981–990.

Executive Committee for the Asymptomatic Carotid Atherosclerosis Study. 1995. "Endarterectomy for Asymptomatic Carotid Artery Stenosis." *JAMA* 273: 1421–28.

Fedoruk J., et. al. 2002. "Rapid on-site Defibrillation Versus Community Program." *Prehospital and Disaster Medicine* 17: 102–06.

Fergusson, Dean, et. al. 2005. "Association Between Suicide Attempts and Selective Serotonin Reuptake Inhibitors: Systematic Review of Randomised Controlled Trials." *British Medical Journal* 330: 396–404.

Fields, Wesley, et. al. 2001. "The Emergency Medical Treatment and Labor Act as a Federal Health Care Safety Net Program." *Academic Emergency Medicine* 8: 1064–69.

Flather, M., et. al. "Long-term ACE-inhibitor Therapy in Patients with Heart Failure or Left-ventricular Dysfunction: a Systematic Overview of Data from Individual Patients." *Lancet* 355: 1578–81.

Flegal, Katherine, et. al. 2005. "Excess Deaths Associated with Underweight, Overweight and Obesity." *JAMA* 293: 1861–1867.

Flum, D., et. al. 2005. "Early Mortality Among Medicare Beneficiaries Underrgoing Bariatric Surgical Procedures." *JAMA* 294: 1903–08.

Fontanarosa, Phil. 2004. "Postmarketing Surveillance—Lack of Vigilance, Lack of Trust. *JAMA* 292: 2647–50.

Ford, Earl, et. al. 2005. "The Prevalence of High Intake of Vitamin E From the Use of Supplements Among U.S. Adults." *Annals of Internal Medicine* 143: 116–20.

Frances, A. 1994. "Foreword," In *Philosophical Perspectives on Psychiatric Diagnostic Classification*, edited by J. Sadler, et al., Baltimore MD: Johns Hopkins University Press.

Francome, Colin, and Wendy Savage. 1993. "Caesarean Section in Britain and the United States 12% or 24%: Is Either the Right Rate?" *Social Science and Medicine* 37: 1199–1218,.

Freed, Curt, et. al. 2001. "Transplantation of Embryonic Dopamine Neurons for Severe Parkinson's Disease." *New England Journal of Medicine* 344: 710–719.

Freedman, Robert. 2003. "Schizophrenia." *New England Journal of Medicine* 349: 1738–49.

Gabbard, Glen. 2004. *The Psychology of the Sopranos*. New York, Basic Books.

Gambone, J., R. Reiter and S. Hagey. 1993. "Clinical Outcomes in Gynecology: Hysterectomy. *Current Problems in Obstetrics, Gynecology and Fertility* 16: 141–66.

———. et. al. 1990. "The Impact of Quality Assurance Process on the Frequency and Confirmation Rate of Hysterectomy." *American Journal of Obstetrics and Gynecology* 163: 545–50.

Gawande, Atul. 2004. "Casualties of War—Military Care for the Wounded from Iraq and Afghanistan. *New England Journal of Medicine* 351: 2471–2475.

Gendler, T. 2000. *Thought Experiment: On the Power and Limits of Imaginary Cases*. New York: Garland.

Glass, Richard. 2004. "Treatment of Adolescents with Major Depression." *JAMA* 292: 861–3.

Gold, M., et. al. 1996. *Cost Effectiveness in Health and Medicine*. New York: Oxford University Press.

Goodman, Stephen. 2002. "Editorial: The Mammography Dilemma: A Crisis for Evidence Based Medicine?" *Annals of Internal Medicine* 137: 363–364.

Goodson, William and Dan Moore. 2002. "Causes of Physician Delay in the Diagnosis of Breast Cancer." *Archives of Internal Medicine* 162: 1343–1348.

Goodwin, James, et. al. 1987. "The Effects of Marital Status on Stage, Treatment, and Survival of Cancer Patients." *JAMA* 258: 3125–30.

Goodwin, Pamela. 2004. "Support Groups in Breast Cancer: When a Negative Result is Positive." *Journal of Clinical Oncology* 22: 4244–46.

———. et. al. 2001. "The Effect of Group Psychosocial Support on Survival in Metastatic Breast Cancer." *New England Journal of Medicine* 345: 1719–26.

Goozner, Merrill. 2004. "Overdosed and Oversold." *New York Times*, December 21.

———. 2004. *"The $800 Million Dollar Pill.* Berkeley: University of California Press.

Gordon, Paul and Janet Senf. 1999. "Is the Annual Complete Physical Examination Necessary?" *Archives of Internal Medicine* 159, 909–910.

Gorman, James. 2004. "The Altered Human is Already Here." *New York Times*, April 6.

Gouldner, Alvin. 1968. "The Sociologist as Partisan: Sociology and the Welfare State." *The American Sociologist* 3: 103–116.

Goy, J. J. 1998. "Intracoronary Stenting." *Lancet* 351: 1943–9.

Grady, Denise. 2003. "Study Finds New Risk in Hormone Therapy." *New York Times*, July 25.

Green, Penelope, et. al. 2001. "The Powerful Placebo: Doubting the Doubters." *Advances in Mind-Body Medicine* 17: 298–307.

Guallar, Eliseo, et. al. 2005. *"Annus horribilis* for Vitamin E." *Annals of Internal Medicine* 143: 143–45.

Haber, Daniel. 2002. "Prophylactic Oophorectomy to Reduce the Risk of Ovarian Breast Cancer in Carriers of BRCA Mutations. *New England Journal of Medicine* 346: 1660–-63.

Haggard, William. 1922. "The Unnecessary Operation." *Surgical Gynecology and Obstetrics* 35: 820.

Hahn, Robert. 1999. "The Nocebo Phenomenon: Scope and Foundations." Pp. 56–76. In *The Placebo Effect,* edited by Ann Harrington, Cambridge: Harvard University Press.

Hammonds, Evelynn. 1999. *Childhood's Deadly Scourge: The Campaign to Control Diphtheria in New York City, 1880–1930.* Baltimore, MD: Johns Hopkins Press.

Han, Paul. 1997. "Historical Changes in the Objectives of the Periodic Health Examination." *Annals of Internal Medicine* 126: 910–917.

Harrington, Ann. 1999. "Introduction." Pp. 1–11 in *The Placebo Effect,* edited by Ann Harrington. Cambridge, MA: Harvard University Press.

Harris, A., et. al. 2002. "Murder and Medicine: the Lethality of Criminal Assault 1960–1999. *Homicide Studies* 6: 128–66.

Harris, Gardiner. 2004. "Study Says Drug's Dangers Were Apparent Years Ago." *New York Times*, November 5.

———. 2004. "FDA Panel Urges Stronger Warning on Antidepressants." *New York Times*, September 15.

———. 2005. "FDA is Advised to Let Pain Pills Stay on the Market." *New York Times*, February 19.

———. 2005. "Drug Makers are Still Giving Gifts to Doctors, FDA Official Says." *New York Times*, March 4.

Harris, A. and Alex Berenson 2005. "10 Voters on Panel Packing Pain Pills had Industry Ties." *New York Times*, February 25.

Harris, R., and L. Kissinger. 2002. "Routinely Teaching Breast Self-examination is Dead. What Does This Mean?" *Journal of the National Cancer Institute* 94: 1420–1421.

Healy, David. 1997. *The Antidepressant Era.* Cambridge, MA: Harvard University Press.

———. 2004. *Let Them Eat Prozac.* New York: New York University Press.

Heart Outcomes Prevention Evaluation Study Investigators. 2000. "Effects of an Angiotensin-converting Enzyme Inhibitor, Ramipril, on Cardiovascular Events in High-risk Patients." *New England Journal of Medicine* 342: 145–53.

The Heart Outcomes Prevention Evaluation Study Investigators. 2000. "Vitamin E Supplementation and Cardiovascular Stents in High-risk Patients. *New England Journal of Medicine* 342: 154–160.

Hedley, Allison, et al. 2004. "Prevalence of Overweight and Obesity Among US Children, Adolescents, and Adults, 1999–2002. *JAMA* 291: 2847–2850.

Heller, Richard, et. al. 2003. "Implementing Guidelines in Primary Care: Can Population Impact Measures Help?" *BMC Public Health* 3: 1–7.

Himmelstein, P. H., et al. 1996. "U.S. Emergency Department Costs: No Emergency." *American Journal of Public Health* 86: 1527–31.

Holder, Angela. 1970. "Unnecessary Surgery." *JAMA* 213: 1755–6.

———. 1972. "Recent Decisions on Unnecessary Surgery." *JAMA* 222: 1593–4.

———. 1975. "Unnecessary Surgery." *JAMA* 232: 1059–60.

Holmes, T., and R. Rahe. 1967. "The Social Readjustment Rating Scale," *Journal of Psychosomatic Research* 11: 213–23.

Honigfeld, G., et. al. , "Reducing Clozapine-related Morbidity and Mortality. *Journal of Clinical Psychiatry* 59 (suppl 3): 3–7.

HOPE and HOPE-TOO Trial Investigators. 2005. "Effects of Long-term Vitamin E Supplementation on Cardiovascular Events and Cancer." *JAMA* 293: 1338–48.

Horowitz, Tamara and Gerald J. Massey, (eds.). 1991. *Thought Experiments in Science and Philosophy.* Savage, MD: Rowman & Littlefield, Inc.

Horton, Richard. 2004. "Vioxx, the Implosion of Merck, and Aftershocks at the FDA." *Lancet* 364: 1995–6.

Houts, Arthur. 2002. "Discovery, Invention, and the Expansion of the Modern *Diagnostic and Statistical Manuals of Mental Disorders.* " In *Rethinking the DSM,* edited by L. Beutler and Mary Malik, Washington, DC: American Psychological Association.

Howard, Barbara, et. al. 2006. "Low Fat Dietary Pattern and Risk of Cardiovascular Disease." *JAMA* 295: 655–66.

Humphry, Linda, et. al. 2002. "Breast Cancer Screening: A Summary of the Evidence for the U.S. Preventive Services Task Force." *Annals of Internal Medicine* 137: 347–367.

Hunsicker, Lawrence. 1990. "Editorial. A Survival Advantage for Renal Transportation. *New England Journal of Medicine* 341: 1762–63.

Hurst, M., and P. Summey. 1984. "Childbirth and Social Class: the Case of Cesarean Delivery." *Social Science and Medicine* 18: 621–31.

Husum, H. 1999. "Effects of Early Prehospital Life Support to War Injured: The Battle of Jalalabad, Afghanistan." *Prehospital and Disaster Medicine* 14: 75–80.

Huyler, Frank. 1999. *The Blood of Strangers: Stories from Emergency Medicine.* Berkeley, CA: University of California Press.

Illich, Ivan. 1976. *Medical Nemesis.* New York: Pantheon.

Institute of Medicine, Division of Health Care Services, Committee on Quality of Health Care Services in America. 1999. *To Err is Human: Building a Safer Health Care System.* Washington, DC, National Academy Press.

Ioannidis, John. 2005. "Contradicted and Initially Stronger Effects in Highly Cited Research," *JAMA* 294: 218–28.

———. et. al. 2001. "Accuracy and Clinical Effect of Out-Of-Hospital Electrocardiography in the Diagnosis of Acute Cardiac Ischemia: a Meta-analysis." *Annals of Emergency Medicine* 37: 461–68.

Jackson, P., et. al. 2001. "Statins for Primary Prevention: At What Coronary Risk is Safety Assured?" *British Journal of Clinical Pharmacology and Therapeutics* 52: 439–46.

Jacobs, Alice. 1999. "Coronary Stents: Have They Fulfilled Their Promise?" *New England Journal of Medicine* 341: 2005–6.

Jasanoff, Sheila, Gerald Markle, Trevor Pinch and James Petersen. 2001. *A Handbook of Science and Technology Studies* 2d ed. (Beverly Hills, CA: Sage Publications.

Jemal, A., et. al. 2005. "Trends in Leading Causes of Death in the United States, 1970–2002." *JAMA* 294: 1255–1299.

Jern, Helen. 1973. *Hormone Therapy of the Menopause and Aging.* Springfield, IL: Charles C. Thomas.

Johnson, A. 1994. "Surgery as Placebo." *Lancet* 344: 114042.

Juni, Peter, et. al. 2004. "Risk of Cardiovascular Events and Rofecoxib: Cumulative Meta-analysis." *Lancet* 364: 2021–29.

Jureidini, Jon, et. al. 2004. "TADS Study Raises Concerns." *British Medical Journal* 329: 1343–44.

Kapchuk, Ted. 1998. "Powerful Placebo: The Dark Side of the Randomized Controlled Trial." *Lancet* 351: 1722–25.

———. 2002. "The Placebo Effect in Alternative Medicine: Can The Performance of a Healing Effect Have Clinical Significance?" *Annals of Internal Medicine* 136: 817–25.

Kauff, N., et. al. 2002. "Risk-reducing Salpingo-oophorectomy in Carriers of BRCA1 or BRCA2 Mutations. *New England Journal of Medicine* 346: 1609-15.

Keating, N., et. al. 1999. "Use of Hormone Replacement Therapy by Postmenopausal Women in the United States. *Annals of Internal Medicine* 130: 545–53.

Keefe, R., et. al. 1999. "The Effects of Atypical Antipsychotic Drugs on Neurocognitive Impairment in Schizophrenia: A Review and Meta-analysis." *Schizophrenia Bulletin* 25: 201–22.

Kelly, Judith, et. al. 2005. "Recent Trends in Use of Herbal and Other Natural Products." *Archives of Internal Medicine* 165: 281–86.

Kessler, Ronald, et. al. 1994. "Lifetime and 12-month Prevalence of *DSM-III-R* Psychiatric Disorders in the United States: Results From the National Comorbidity Survey." *Archives of General Psychiatry* 51: 8–19.

————. et. al. 1999. "Past-year Use of Outpatient Services for Psychiatric Problems in the National Comorbidity Survey." *American Journal of Psychiatry* 156: 115–23.

Kim, Peter and Alise Reicin. 2005. "Discontinuation of Vioxx." *Lancet* 365: 23.

Kohn, L. T., et. al. *To Error is Human.* Washington, DC National Academy Press.

Kolata, Gina. 2003. "Annual Physical Checkup May Be An Empty Ritual." *New York Times*, August 12.

————. 2003. "There's a Blurry Line Between Rx and O.T.C." *New York Times*, December 23.

————. 2004. "New Studies Cast Doubt on Artery-opening Operations." *New York Times*, March 21, 2004.

————. "Good Pill, Bad Pill: Science Makes it Hard to Decipher." *New York Times*, December 22.

————. 2005. "Panel to Advise Testing Babies for 29 Diseases." *New York Times*, February 25.

Koroukian, S. 1998. "Estimating the Proportion of Unnecessary Cesarean Sections in Ohio Using Birth Certificate Data. *Journal of Clinical Epidemiology* 51: 1327–1334.

Kuhn, Thomas. 1962. *The Structure of Scientific Revolutions.* University of Chicago Press.

————. 1977. "A Function for Thought Experiments." Pp. 240–266. In *The Essential Tension*, edited by Thomas Kuhn, Chicago: University of Chicago Press.

Kunitz, Stephen. 1987. "Explanations and Ideologies of Mortality Patterns." *Population and Development Review* 13: 380.

————. 1991. "The Personal Physician and the Decline in Mortality." P. 248. In *The Decline of Mortality in Europe*, edited by R. Schofield, D. Reher and A. Bideau. Oxford: Clarendon Press.

LaCaze, Marguerite. 2002. *The Analytic Imagery*. Ithaca: Cornell University Press.

Lafata, Jennifer, et. al. 2004. "The Economic Impact of False-positive Cancer screens." *Cancer Epidemiology Biomarkers and Prevention* 13: 2126–32.

Lane, Christine. 2002. "The Annual Physical Examination: Needless Ritual or Necessary Routine?" Editorial. *Annals of Internal Medicine* 136: 701–703.

Lange, Richard and L. David Hollis. 1998. "Use and Overuse of Angiography and Revascularization for Acute Coronary Syndromes." *New England Journal of Medicine* 338: 1838–9.

Langewitz, Wolf, et. al. 2002. "Spontaneous Talking Time at Start of Consultation in Outpatient Clinic: Cohort Study." *British Medical Journal* 325: 682–683.

Lazarou, Jason, Bruce H. Pomeranz and Paul Corey. 1998. "Incidence of Adverse Drug Reactions in Hospitalized Patients: A Meta-analysis of Prospective Studies." *JAMA* 279: 1200–1205.

Leaque, D. 2003. "Endometrial Ablation as an Alternative to Hysterectomy." *AORN Journal* 77: 322–338.

Lee, et. al. 1984. "Confirmation of the Pre-operative Diagnosis for Hysterectomy." *American Journal of Obstetrics and Gynecology* 150: 283–87.

Lee, I-Min, et. al. 2005. "Vitamin E in the Primary Prevention of Cardiovascular Disease and Cancer." *JAMA* 294: 56–65.

Lerman, Caryn, et. al. 1991. "Psychological and Behavioral Implications of Abnormal Mammograms." *Annals of Internal Medicine* 114: 657–661.

Letourneau, Charles. 1953. "The Legal and Moral Aspects of 'Unnecessary Surgery.'" *Hospitals* 27:82.

Levine, Sol, et. al. 1983. "Does Medical Care Do Any Good?" Chapter 18. In *Handbook of Health, Health Care and the Health Professionals*, edited by David Mechanic. New York: Free Press.

Lewis, David. 2002. "Atypical Antipsychotic Medications and the Treatment of Schizophrenia." *British Journal of Psychiatry* 159: 177–9.

Lichtenstein, Alice and Robert Russell. 2005. "Essential Nutrients: Food or Supplements?" *JAMA* 294: 351–58.

Lillberg, Kirsi, et. al. 2003. "Stressful Life Events and Risk of Breast Cancer in 10,808 Women: A Cohort Study." *American Journal of Epidemiology* 157: 415–23.

MacLean, Catherine, et. al. 2006. "Effects of Omega-3 Fatty Acids on Cancer Risk." *JAMA* 295: 403–415.

Maier, J., and J. Maloni. 1997. "Nurse Advocacy for Selective Versus Routine Episiotomy." *Journal of Obstetric, Gynecologic and Neonatal Nursing.* 26: 155–61.

Mangione, Salvatore and Linda Neiman. 1997. "Cardiac Auscultatory Skills of Internal Medicine and Family Practice Trainees." *JAMA* 278: 717–722.

Markle, Gerald and Daryl Chubin. 1987. "Consensus Development in Medicine: The Liver Transplant Controversy." *Milbank Quarterly* 65: 1–24.

Markle, Gerald and James Petersen. 1980. *Science, Politics and Cancer: The Laetrile Phenomenon.* American Association for the Advancement of Science Selected Symposia Series, Boulder, CO: Westview Press.

Markle, Gerald and Frances B. McCrea. 1990. "Forgetting and Remembering: Bitburg and the Social Construction of History." *Perspectives on Social Problems* 2: 143–159.

Marshall, Ian and Danah Zohar. 1997. *Who's Afraid of Schrodinger's Cat?* New York: William Morrow.

McCrea, Frances. 1983. "The Politics of Menopause: The 'Discovery' of a Deficiency Disease." *Social Problems*, 31, no. 1: 111–123.

McCrea, Frances. and Gerald Markle. 1984. "The Estrogen Replacement Controversy in the United States and Great Britain: Different Answers to the Same Question?" *Social Studies of Science*, 14, no. 1: 1–26.

McGinnis, J., and William Foege. "Editorial: The Immediate vs the Important." *JAMA* 291: 1363–64.

McKeown, Thomas. 1979. *The Role of Medicine: Dream, Mirage or Nemesis.* London: Nuffield Provincial Hospitals Trust 1976. Princeton, NJ: Princeton University Press.

———, 1978. "Fertility, Mortality and Causes of Death." *Population Studies* 32: 535.

McKinley, John. "A Case for Refocusing Upstream: the Political Economy of Illness." In *Applying Behavioral Science to Cardiovasuclar Risk.* NY: American Heart Association.

Mckinley, John and Sonja McKinley. 1977. "The Questionable Contribution of Medical Measures to the Decline of Mortality in the United States in the Twentieth Century." *Milbank Memorial Fund Quarterly* (Summer): 405–428.

Malmsheimer, Richard. *Doctors Only: The Evolving Image of the American Physician.* New York: Greenwood Press.

Matheson, J., and D. Figgit. 2001. "Rofecoxib: A Review of its Use in the Management of Osteoarthritis, Acute Pain and Rheumatoid Arthritis." *Drugs* 61: 833–65.

Matthew, A., and B. Martinez. 2004. "E-mails Suggest Merck knew Vioxx's Dangers at Early Stage." *Wall Street Journal*, November 1, p. A–1.

Mathews, Ella. 2005. "Response to 'A Controversy not Far Enough.'" *British Medical Journal* 329: 1397.

Mayberg, Marc and Richard Winn. 1995. "Endarterectomy for Asymptomatic Carotid Artery Stenosis. An Editorial. *JAMA* 273: 1459–61.

Meckel, Richard. 1990. *Save the Babies: American Public Health Reform and the Prevention of Infant Mortality.* Baltimore, MD: Johns Hopkins Press.

Mehta, J. 1997. "Intake of Antioxidants Among American Cardiologists." *American Journal of Cardiology* 79: 1558–60.

Meier, Barry. 2004. "Medicine Fueled by Marketing Intensified Trouble for Pain Pills." *New York Times*, December 19.

Melmed, Raphael. 2001. *Mind, Body, and Medicine.* New York: Oxford University Press.

Mctlay, Joshua, et. al. 1998. "National Trends in the Use of Antibiotics by Primary Care Physicians for Adult Patients With Cough." *Archives of Internal Medicine* 158: 1813–1818.

Miller, Anthony, et. al. 2002. "The Canadian National Breast Screening Study-1: Breast Cancer Mortality After 11 to 16 Years of Follow-up." *Annals of Internal Medicine* 137: 305–315.

Miller, N. 1946. "Hysterectomy: Therapeutic Necessity or Surgical Racket?" *American Journal of Obstetrics and Gynecology* 51: 804–10.

Mishara, A., and T. Goldberg. 2004 "A Meta-analysis and Critical Review of the Effects of Conventional Neuroleptic Treatment on Cognition in Schizophrenia: Opening a Closed Book." *Biological Psychiatry* 55: 1013–22.

MMWR. 2001. "New York City Department of Health Response to Terrorist Attack, September 11, 2001." *Morbidity and Mortality Weekly Report* 50: 821–2.

Moerman, Daniel and Wayne Jonas. 1976. "Deconstructing the Placebo Effect and Finding the Meaning Response." *Annals of Internal Medicine* 136: 471–76.

Mokdad, Ali, et. al. 2004. "Actual Cause of Death in the United States, 2000." *JAMA* 291: 1238–45.

Morel, Marie-France. 1991. "The Care of Children: The Influence of Medical Innovation and the Medical Institutions on Infant Mortality, 1750–1914." Pp. 196–219. In *The Decline of Mortality in Europe*, edited by R. Schofield, D. Reher and A. Bideau. Oxford: Clarendon Press.

Morris, C., et. al. 2003. "Routine Vitamin Supplementation to Prevent Cardiovascular Disease: A Summary of Evidence for the US Preventive Services Task Force. *Annals of Internal Medicine* 239: 56–70.

Morris, David. 1999. "Placebo, Pain and Belief: A Biocultural Model." Pp. 187–207. In *The Placebo Effect,* edited by Ann Harrington, Cambridge: Harvard University Press.

Mosely, J., et. al. 2002. "A Controlled Trial of Arthroscopic Surgery for Osteoarthritis of the Knee." *New England Journal of Medicine* 347: 81–88.

Moyers, Bill 1993. *Healing and the Mind.* New York: Doubleday.

Mukherjee, D., et. al. 2001. "Risk of Cardiovascular Events Associated with Selective COX-2 Inhibitors." *JAMA* 286: 954–9.

Murray, D., et. al. 1986. "Systematic Risk Factor Screening and Education: A Community-wide Approach to the Prevention of Coronary Heart Disease." *Preventive Medicine* 15: 661–672.

Myers, R. B. 1998. "Pre-hospital Management of Acute Myocardial Infarction: Electrocardiogram Acquisition and Interpretation, and Thrombolysis by Pre-hospital Care Providers." *The Canadian Journal of Cardiology* 14: 1231–40.

Nagourney, Eric. 2003. "Doctors Use Casino as Lab to Test Secondhand Smoke." *New York Times*, December 23.

National Association of Chain Drug Stores. 2003. *The Chain Pharmacy Industry Profile.* Alexandria, VA: National Association of Chain Drug Stores.

National Center for Complementary and Alternative Medicine. 2004. *Mind-Body Medicine: An Overview.* Bethesda, MD: National Institutes of Health.

National Institutes of Health, NIH News Release. 1997. "NIH Panel Issues Consensus Statement on Acupuncture," November 5.

National Institute of Mental Health. 2002. *Depression*. Bethesda, MD: #02–3561.

———. 2001. *The Numbers Count: Mental Disorders in America*. Bethesda, MD: 01–4584.

———. *Schizophrenia*. Bethesda, MD.

Neale, A., et. al. 1986. "Marital Status, Delay in Seeking Treatment, and Survival from Breast Cancer." *Social Science and Medicine* 23: 305–312.

Nelson, Heidi, et. al. 2002. "Postmenopausal Hormone Replacement Therapy for the Primary Prevention of Chronic Conditions: A Summary of Evidence for the U.S. Preventive Task Force." Agency for Health Care Research and Quality.

New England Journal of Medicine. 2004. "Looking Back on the Millennium in Medicine." *New England Journal of Medicine* 342: 42–49.

New York Times. 2004. "What the Body Knows." *New York Times*, March 4.

Nichols, Graham, et. al. 1999. "A Cumulative Meta-analysis of the Effectiveness of Defibrillator-capable Emergency Medical Services for Victims of Out-of-hospital Cardiac Arrest." *Annals of Emergency Medicine* 34: 517-25.

Norton, John. 1991. "Thought Experiments in Einstein's Work." Pp. 129–144. In *Thought Experiments in Science and Philosophy*. edited by Tamara Horowitz and Gerald Massey. Savage, MD: Rowman & Littlefield.

Numbers, Ronald. "The History of American Medicine: A Field in Ferment." *Reviews in American History* 10: 245–263.

O'Connor, Michael. 1998. "The Role of the Television Drama *ER* in the Medical Student's Life: Entertainment or Socialization?" *JAMA* 280: 854–855.

Organization for Economic Cooperation and Development. 2004. *OECD Health Data, 2004. A Comparative Analysis of 29 Countries*. Paris: OECD.

Office of Technology Assessment. 1983 *The Impact of Randomized Clinical Trials on Health Policy and Medical Practice*. Washington, D.C.: U.S. Government Printing Office.

Olson, F. 1999. "No Room at the Inn: A Snapshot of an American Emergency Room." *Stanford Law Review* 46: 449–501.

Paola, Robert and Ronald Morton. 2006. "Proven and Unproven Therapy for Benign Hyperstatic Hyperplasia." *New England Journal of Medicine* 354: 632–33.

Parker, Amy, et. al. 2006. "Implications of a 2005 Measles Outbreak in Indiana For Sustained Elimination of Measles in the United States." *New England Journal of Medicine* 355: 447–55.

Pauly, M. 1979. "What is Unnecessary Surgery?" *Milbank Memorial Fund Quarterly* 57: 95–117.

Pasko, Thomas and B. Seidman, (eds.) 2003. *Physician Characteristics and Distribution in the United States*. Chicago: American Medical Association.

Pear, Robert. 2004. "Americans Relying More on Prescription Drugs, Report Says." *New York Times*, December 3.

Petersen, James, and Gerald Markle. 1981. "Expansion of Conflict in Cancer Controversies." PP. 151–169. In *Research in Social Movements, Conflicts and Change*, edited by Louis Kriesberg. Greenwich, CT: JAI Press.

Phillips, D., et. al. 1993. "Psychology and Survival." *Lancet* 344: 1142–45.

Pickering, T.G., et. al. 1988. "How Common is White Coat Hypertension?" *JAMA* 259: 225–228.

Pignone, Michael, et. al. 2002. "Cost-effectiveness Analysis of Colorectal Cancer Screening: A Systematic Review for the U.S. Preventive Services Task Force." *Annals of Internal Medicine* 137: 96–104.

Pilling, S., et. al. 2002. "Psychological Treatments in Schizophrenia: II. Meta-analysis of Randomized Controlled Trials of Social Skills Training and Cognitive Remediation." *Psychological Medicine* 32: 783–91.

Pincus, Harold, et. al. 1999. "Psychiatric Patients and Treatments in 1997." *Archives of General Psychiatry* 56: 441–49.

Pitt, Bertram. 2005. "Low Density Lipoprotein Cholesterol in Patients with Stable Heart Disease—Is It Time to Shift our Goals?" *New England Journal of Medicine*, April 7.

Pollack, Andrew. 2005. "Medical Researcher Moves to Sever Ties to Companies." *New York Times*, January 25.

Pope, J. H., et. al. 2000. "Missed Diagnoses of Acute Cardiac Ischemia in the Emergency Department." *New England Journal of Medicine* 342: 1163–70.

Porter, Roy. 1997. *The Greatest Benefit to Mankind*. New York: Norton.

Powles, John. 1974. "On the Limitations of Modern Medicine." Pp. 89–122. In *The Challenges of Community Medicine*, edited by Robert Kane. New York: Springer.

Prentice, Ross, et. al. 2006. "Low-fat Dietary Pattern and Risk of Invasive Breast Cancer." *JAMA* 295: 629–42.

Psaty, Bruce, et. al. 2003. "Health Outcomes Associated with Various Antihypertensive Therapies Used as First-line Agents. *JAMA* 289: 2534–44.

———. 2004. "Potential For Conflict of Interest in the Evaluation of Suspected Adverse Drug Reactions." *JAMA* 292: 2622–31.

Punglia, Rina, et. al. 2003. "Effect of Verification Bias on Screening for Prostate Cancer by Measurement of Prostate Specific Antigen." *New England Journal of Medicine* 349: 335–42.

RAND Corporation. 1987. "Health Services Utilization Study. RAND Report.

Ransohoff, David, et. al. 1983. "Prophylactic Cholecystectomy or Expectant Management for Silent Gallstones." *Annals of Internal Medicine* 99: 199.

Ransohoff, David and Charles McSherry. 1995. "Why are Cholecystectomy Rates Increasing?" *JAMA* 273: 1621–22.

Rea, Thomas, et. al. 2003. "Emergency Medical Services and Mortality from Heart Disease: A Community Study." *Annals of Emergency Medicine* 41: 494–99.

Rebbeck, T., et. al. 2002. "Prophylactic Oophorectomy in Carriers of BRCA1 or BRCA2 Mutations." *New England Journal of Medicine* 346: 1616–22.

Relman, Arnold, and Marcia Angell. 2002. "America's Other Drug Problem." *New Republic*, December 16.

Reston, James. 1971. "Now Let Me Tell You About My Appendectomy in Peking..." *New York Times*, July 26.

Reuben, David. 1969. *Everything You Always Wanted To Know About Sex But Were Afraid To Ask*. New York: David McKay.

Richardson, Lynne, and Ula Hwang. 2001. "Access to Care: A Review of the Emergency Medicine Literature." *Academic Emergency Medicine* 8: 1030–36.

Ridker, Paul and Jose Torres. 2000–2005. "Reported Outcomes in Major Cardiovascular Clinical Trials Funded by For-Profit and Not-For-Profit Organizations, 2000–2005." *JAMA* 295: 2270–2274.

Roberts, A., et. al. 1993. "The Power of Nonspecific Effects in Medicine and Surgery: Implications for Biological and Psychosocial Treatments." *Clinical Psychology Review* 13: 375–91.

Rosen, George. 1975. *Preventive Medicine in the United States, 1900–1975: Trends and Interpretations*. New York: History of Science.

Rosenhan, David. 1973. "On Being Sane in Insane Places." *Science* 179: 250–258.

Rutkow, Ira. 1989, "Unnecessary Surgery." Pp. 333–351, In *Socioeconomics of Surgery*, edited by Ira Rutkow, St. Louis: Mosby.

———. 1989. "Surgical Operations and Manpower: Can Technical Proficiency be Manufactured?" In *Socioeconomics*, edited by Ira Rutkow. St. Louis: Mosby.

Sacks, Frank. 2001. "Lipid-lowering Therapy in Acute Coronary Syndromes." *JAMA* 285: 1758–60.

Sacks, Oliver. 1995. *An Anthropologist on Mars*. P. xvi. New York: Alfred A. Knopf.

Sakala, Carol.1993. "Medically Unnecessary Cesarean Section Births: Introduction to a Symposium." *Social Science and Medicine* 37: 1177–98.

Sanders, Arthur and Gordon Ewy. 2005. "Cardiopulmonary Resuscitation in the Real World: When Will the Guidelines Get the Message?" *JAMA* 293: 363–65.

Santry, Heena, et. al. 2005. "Trends in Bariatric Surgical Procedures." *JAMA* 294: 1909–17.

Sargent, Richard, et. al. 2004. "Reduced Incidence of Admissions for Myocardial Infarction Associated with Public Smoking Ban: Before and After Study. *British Medical Journal* 328: 977–980.

Saul, Stephanie. 2005. "More Celebreties Finding Roles as Antidepressant Advocates. *New York Times*, March 21.

Schaffer, J., and A. Word. 2002. "Hysterectomy—Still a Useful Operation." *New England Journal of Medicine* 347: 1360–62.

Scheff, Thomas. 1966. *Being Mentally Ill*. Chicago: Aldine.

Schernhammer, E., et. al. 2004. "Job Stress and Breast Cancer Risk: The Nurses Health Study." *American Journal of Epidemiology* 160: 1079–86.

Schonfield, R. 1991. The Decline of Mortality in Europe. Oxford: Clarendon Press.

Schwartz, Gregory, et. al. 2001. "Effects of Atorvastatin on Early Recurrent Ischemic Events in Acute Coronary Syndromes." *JAMA* 285: 1711–18.

Scott, J., et. al. 2001. "Antibiotic Use in Acute Respiratory Infections and the Ways Patients Pressure Physicians for a Prescription." *Journal of Family Practice* 50: 853–858.

Scully, James and Joshua Wilk. 2003. "Selected Characteristics and Data of Psychiatrists in the United States, 2001–2002." *Academic Psychiatry* 27: 247–51.

Selzer, Richard. 1982. *Letters to a Young Doctor*. NY: Simon & Schuster.

Sever, P. S., et. al. 2003. "Prevention of Coronary and Stroke Events with Atorvastatin in Hypertensive Patients Who Have Average or Lower-Than-Average Cholesterol Concentration, in the Anglo-Scandinavian Cardiac Outcomes Trial (ASCOT): A Multi-center, Randomized Controlled Trial." *Lancet* 361: 1149–1158.

Shapiro, Arthur and Elaine Shapiro. 1997. *The Powerful Placebo*. Baltimore, MD: Johns Hopkins University Press.

Sharpe, Virginia and Alan Faden. 1998. *Medical Harm*. Cambridge: Cambridge University Press.

Shearer, E. 1993. "Cesarean Section: Medical Benefits and Costs." *Social Science and Medicine* 37: 1223–31.

Shelton, Richard, et. al. 2001. "Effectiveness of St. John's Wort in Major Depression." *JAMA* 285: 1978–86.

Shepard J., et. al. 2002. "Pravastatin in Elderly Individuals at Risk of Vascular Disease (PROSPER): A Randomized Clinical Trial." *Lancet* 360:1623–30.

Shumaker, S., et. al. 2003. "Estrogen Plus Progestin and the Incidence of Dementia and Mild Cognitive Impairment in Postmenopausal Women: The Women's Helath Initiative Memory Study: A Randomized Controlled Trial." *Journal of the American Medical Association* 289: 2651–62.

Simonsen, Lone, et. al. 2005. "Impact of Influenza Vaccination on Seasonal Mortality in the U.S. Elderly Population." *Archives of Internal Medicine* 165: 265–72.

Sonnenberg, Amnon, et. al. 2000. "Cost-Effectiveness of Colonoscopy in Screening for Colorectal Cancer." *Annals of Internal Medicine* 133: 573–584.

Sorensen, Roy. 1992. *Thought Experiments*. New York: Oxford.

Sox, Harold. 2002. "Editorial: Screening Mammography for Younger Women: Back to Basics." *Annals of Internal Medicine* 137: 361–362.

Spiegel, David, 2004. "Placebos in Practice." *British Medical Journal* 329: 927–8.

———. 2001. "Mind Matters—Group Therapy and Survival in Breast Cancer." *New England Journal of Medicine* 345: 1767–8.

———. 1993. "Social Support: How Friends, Family, and Groups Can Help." Pp. 332–349. In *Mind Body Medicine*, edited by Daniel Goleman and Joel Gurin. Yonkers, NY: Consumer Report Books.

————, et. al. 1989. "Effect of Psychosocial Treatment on Survival of Patients with Metastatic Breast Cancer." *Lancet* 2: 888–91.

Spiegel, David and Griese-Davis, Janine. 2003. "Depression and Cancer: Mechanism and Disease Progression." *Biological Psychiatry* 54: 269–82.

Spiro, Howard. 1999. "Clinical Reflections on the Placebo Phenomenon." Pp. 37–55. In *The Placebo Effect*, edited by Ann Harrington. Cambridge, MA: Harvard University Press.

Starr, Paul. 1982. *The Social Transformation of American Medicine*. New York: Basic Books.

Stephens, M., et. al. 2000. "The Maternal Perspective on Prenatal Ultrasound." *Journal of Family Practice* 49: 601–604.

Stiell, I. G., et. al. 1999. "Improved Out-Of-Hospital Cardiac Survival Through the Inexpensive Optimization of an Existing Defibrillation Program: OPALS Study Phase II." *JAMA* 281: 1175–81.

Strandberg, T., et. al. 2004. "Mortality and incidence of cancer during 10-year follow-up of the Scandinavian Simvastatin Survival Study (4S)." *Lancet* 364: 771–7.

Steinbrook, Robert. 2006. "Imposing Personal Responsibility for Health." *New England Journal of Medicine* 55: 753–56.

Strom, Brian. 2005. "Statins and Over-the-Counter Availability." *New England Journal of Medicine* 352:1403–05.

Szasz, Thomas. 1970. *Ideology and Insanity*. Garden City, NY: Anchor Books.

————. 2004. *Pharmacy*. Westport, CT: Praeger.

————. 2004. "It is More Controversial to Prescribe Anti-depressants Than Not." *British Medical Journal* 329: 1397.

Taylor, Todd. 2001. "Threats to the Health Care Safety Net." *Academic Emergency Medicine* 8: 1080–87.

Therapeutics Initiative. 2003. "Do Statins Have a Role in Primary Prevention?" *Therapeutics Letter* 48: June.

Thomas, David, et. al. 2002. "Randomized Trial of Breast Self-examination in Shanghai: Final Results." *Journal of the National Cancer Institute* 94: 1445–1457.

Thomas, Lewis. 1975. *The Lives of a Cell: Notes of a Biology Watcher*. New York: Bantam Books.

Timimi, Sami. 2004. "Rethinking Childhood Depression." *British Medical Journal* 329: 1394–96.

———. "It is More Controversial to Prescribe Anti-depressants Than Not."

Topol, Eric. 2004. "Good Riddance to a Bad Drug." *New York Times*, October 2.

———. 2004. "Failing the Public Health—Rofecoxib, Merck, and the FDA." *New England Journal of Medicine* 351: 1707–09.

Treatment for Adolescents with Depression Study (TADS) Team. "Fluoxetine, Cognitive-Behavioral Therapy, and Their Combination for Adolescents with Depression." *JAMA* 292: 807–20.

Troyer, Ronald and Gerald Markle. 1983. *Cigarettes: The Battle Over Smoking.* New Brunswick, NJ: Rutgers University Press.

Tuller, David. 2004. "Seeking a Fuller Picture of Statins." *New York Times*, July 20.

Turner, J., et. al. 1994. "The Importance of Placebo Effect in Pain Treatment and Research." *JAMA* 271:1609–14.

Tussing, A., and Martha Worrowycz. 1993. "The Effect of Physician Characteristics on Clinical Behavior: Cesarean Section in New York State. *Social Science and Medicine* 37: 1251–60.

Ueshima, K., et. al. 2004. "Is Angiotensin-Converting Enzyme Inhibitor Useful in a Japanese Population for Secondary Prevention after Acute Myocardial Infarction? A final Report of the Japanese Acute Myocardial Infarction Prospective (JAMP) study." *American Heart Journal* 148: e8.

U.S. Bureau of the Census. 2005. *Infant Mortality and Life Expectancy for Selected Countries, 2005.* Washington, DC: U.S. Government Printing Office.

U. S. Congress. 1976. House Committee on Interstate and Foreign Commerce. Subcommittee on Oversight and Investigation. "Cost and Quality of Health Care: Unnecessary Surgery." Washington, D.: U.S. Government Printing Office.

U.S. Department of Health and Human Services. 1989. Health Care Financing Administration, *The International Classification of Disease, 9th Revision, ICD—9-CM.* Washington, DC: U.S. Government Printing Office.

———. 1994. National Hospital Ambulatory Medical Care Survey: 1992 Emergency Department Summary. Vital and Health Statistics, Advance Data, 245: 1–12.

———. 2002. "National Hospital Ambulatory Medical Care Survey: 2000 Emergency Department Summary. Vital and Health Statistics, Advance Data, April 22, 2002 (#326).

U.S. General Accounting Office. 1993. "Emergency Departments: Unevenly Affected by Growth and Change in Patient Use." No. B-251319. Washington, DC: U.S. Government Printing Office.

U.S. Preventive Services Task Force. 1989. *Guide to Clinical Preventive Services: An Assessment of the Effectiveness of 169 Interventions.* Baltimore, MD: Williams & Wilkins..

———. 1996. *Guidelines to Clinical Preventive Services*, 2nd ed. Baltimore, MD: Williams & Wilkins.

———. 2002. "Screening for Breast Cancer: Recommendations and Rationale." *Annals of Internal Medicine* 137:344–346.

Vickers, A. 2004. "Alternative Cancer Cures" "Unproven" or "Disproven"? *CA: A Journal for Clinicians* 54: 110–118.

Vrecer, M., et. al. 2003. "Use of Statins in Primary and Secondary Prevention of Coronary Heart Disease and Ischemic Strokes: Meta-analysis of Randomized Trials." *International Journal of Clinical Pharmacology and Therapeutics* 41: 567–77.

Wahlbeck, K., et. al. 2001. "Dropout Rates in Randomized Antipsychotic Drug Trials." *Psychopharmacology* 155: 230–33.

Wainwright, S., et. al. 1999. "Cardiovascular Mortality—the Hidden Peril of Heat Waves." *Prehospital and Disaster Medicine* 14: 222–31.

Weijer, C. 2002. "I need a Placebo Like I Need a Hole in the Head." *Journal of Law and Medical Ethics* 30: 69.

Wellbery, Caroline. 1997. "Editorial: Are We Prescribing too Many Antibiotics?" *American Family Physician* 55 no 5.

Wennberg, David, et. al. 1999. "Pounds of Prevention for Ounces of Cure: Surgery as a Preventive Strategy." *Lancet* 353: S9–S11.

Wennberg, John. 1989. "Small Area Variations and the Practice Style Factor." Pp. 67–91. In *Socioeconomics of Surgery*, edited by Ira Rutkow. St. Louis: Mosby.

Wennberg, J. and M. Cooper (eds.). *The Quality of Medical Care in the United States: A Report on the Medicare Program.* Chicago: American Hospital Publishing.

Whittman, W. 1990. "Natural History of Low-stage Prostate Cancer and the Impact of Early Detection." *Urological Clinical Studies North America* 17: 689–697.

Wik, Lars, et. al. 2005. "Quality of Cardiopulmonary Resuscitation During Out-Of-Hospital Cardiac Arrest." *JAMA* 293: 299–304.

Williams, R. 1996. "The Costs of Visits to Emergency Departments." *New England Journal of Medicine* 334: 642–6.

Wilson, Robert. 1963. *Feminine Forever*. New York: M. Evans.

Wilson, Robert, and Thelma Wilson. 1963. "The Fate of Postmenopausal Women: A Plea for the Maintenance of Adequate Estrogen From Puberty to Grave." *Journal of the American Geriatrics Society* 11: 347–61.

Wolf, Stewart. 1959. "The Pharmacology of Placebos." *Pharmacological Reviews* 2: 689–704.

Wolfe, Bruce, and John Morton. 2005. "Weighing in on Bariatric Surgery." *JAMA* 294: 1960–63.

Wolfe, Robert, et. al. 1999. "Comparison of Mortality in all Patients on Dialysis, Patients on Dialysis Awaiting Transplantation, and Recipients of a First Cadaveric Transplant. *New England Journal of Medicine* 341: 1725–30.

Wolpe, P. 1985. "The Maintenance of Professional Authority: Acupuncture and the American Physician." *Social Problems* 32: 409–424.

Wolsko, P., et. al. 2004. "Use of Mind-body Medical Therapies." *Journal of General Internal Medicine* 19: 43–50.

Women's Health Initiative. 2002. "Risks and Benefits of Estrogen Plus Progestin in Healthy Menopausal Women: Principal Results From the Women's Health Initiative Randomized Controlled Trial." *JAMA* 288: 321–22.

The World Health Organization. 1958. *The First Ten Years*. Geneva: World Health Organization,

Young, G. P., et. al. 1996. "Ambulatory Visits to Hospital Emergency Departments. Patterns and Reasons for Use: 24 Hours in the ED Study Group." *JAMA* 276: 460–65.

Zarin, Deborah, et. al. 1998. "Characterizing Psychiatry with Findings From the 1996 National Survey of Psychiatric Practice." *American Journal of Psychiatry* 115: 397–404.

Ziporyn, Terra. 1988. *Diseases in the Popular American Press: The Case of Diphtheria, Typhoid Fever, and Syphilis, 1870–1920*. New York: Greenwood Press.

Index

227

Made in the USA
Lexington, KY
13 November 2010